D0375689

What Women MUST Know To

Protect Their Daughters

From

Breast Cancer

by
Dr. Sherrill Sellman, N.D.

1st Edition: June 2005

ISBN 0-9750487-4-0

Production & Cover graphics by: G4&Duck Designs

Photo Credit: Dennis Ryan - Melbourne Australia

Australian Distribution: Brumby Book Distributors
                          10 Southfork Drive
                          Kilsyth South, Victoria 3137
                          61 3 9761-5535 voice
                          61 3 9761-7095 fax

Dearest Kathy,

Your love and light are a blessing to this world — and to me!

CJ Sherrill

Contents

Chapter 5
Soy Infant Formulas

Chapter 6

Chapter 7
Doing It Yourself

Dedication

To Karissa,
my "inherited" daughter
but, more importantly,
my soul sister
in this life's journey.

To all
who have lost
a mother, aunt,
sister, daughter
or friend
to breast cancer
and
to the young women
of today and all future
generations of women.
May they be blessed with
the Wisdom and Beauty
of the Feminine
so health, joy, and harmony
will be theirs
forever.

Introduction

Since publishing my first book, *Hormone Heresy - What Women MUST Know About Their Hormones*, my world has totally changed. I have changed careers; I have changed my residence; and I have radically changed many of my ideas concerning women's health. I have embarked on a mission to educate women worldwide about the benefits of holistic approaches to hormonal health and wellbeing.

The more I investigated the many health problems currently facing women, the more committed I have become to disseminating the facts. I have learned that when it comes to hormonal health, there is much that women are not being told. And, often the medical advice and treatment options have been down right dangerous.

It was with mixed feelings that I received the headline news in July 2002 when the largest study ever conducted on HRT, the Women's Health Initiative, abruptly ended three years earlier than expected. The preliminary findings sent shock waves ricocheting around the world. What would cause a massive multi-million dollar study to close its doors? As it turned out, the researchers found an undeniable link between the use of HRT and a significant increase in breast cancer, strokes and blood clots.

On the one hand, I felt a sense of triumph since this was exactly what I had been warning women about for a decade. On the other hand, I felt great sadness for all the millions of women worldwide who suffered and, in some cases, died as a result of being prescribed these drugs.

Since then, numerous studies have confirmed that HRT is, in fact, "a major medical mistake". Therefore, it could be argued that, women using HRT were really the unconsenting guinea pigs in a massive experiment.

Wherever I was invited to present my message – throughout the US, Canada, Australia, the UK and Ireland – women would share their many stories with me. So many women were wrestling with a wide variety of hormonal problems and illnesses. I learned of their frustration with menopausal and perimenopausal symptoms; their battle to save their uteruses and ovaries; their infertility problems; the pain of endometriosis; the fear of osteoporosis and much more. And, of course, I would hear of the many numerous accounts of personal battles being waged against breast cancer.

Along with millions of women, I have always believed that older women were most at risk. You can imagine my shock and horror when I began to meet a growing number of young women who were also fighting this dreaded disease. As tragic as it is, I can accept that the risk of breast cancer increases with age. But, these were women in their 40's, 30's and 20's! At first I couldn't believe it. I initially thought that breast cancer showing up in young women must be some aberration of the norm, a one–in –a-million stroke of bad luck.

But I have since come to realize this is not the case. In fact, for the past several years, I have been talking with more and more of the young breast cancer survivors hearing their stories, they're struggles and their fears.

A corollary to this problem is the epidemic number of hormonal imbalances occurring in young women. These conditions include:

- PMS
- Ovarian cysts
- Polycystic ovaries
- Endometriosis
- Early puberty

- Depression
- Fibroids
- Hypothyroidism
- Fibrocystic breast disease

Why should this be of concern? Because, there is an acknowledged link between these persistent hormonal problems and an increased risk of breast cancer later in life.

After ten years of researching these issues and observing the deteriorating health of young women, I felt it was imperative to raise the alarm. The sad fact is that young women, more than ever before are hormonally out of balance. In this modern day and age, it's hard to find a teenager or young adult, who isn't dealing with some sort of hormonal problem. In fact, such conditions have become so common that many women readily accept them as normal. It is important to understand, however, that PMS, ovarian cysts, endometriosis or polycystic ovaries are not by any stretch of the imagination normal occurrences but rather signs that the body is out of balance. Long-term hormonal imbalances are fertile ground for more serious problems such as breast cancer down the track.

Can I really be so bold as to say that women, especially young women, can be protected from breast cancer? Many people would argue that such a statement exists in the realm of wishful thinking.

And no wonder! If you listen to the American Cancer Society's position on breast cancer, it would certainly affirm the belief that women are, indeed, merely helpless victims being hounded down by a relentless breast cancer monster. With sincere regrets they announced, "At this time, there is no way to prevent breast cancer." The National Cancer Institute is no more helpful. "Breast Cancer is simply not a preventable disease", it states matter-of-factly.

I absolutely do believe that there is much that women can do to protect themselves from breast cancer. And, in addition, we can help protect younger women, our daughters, from ever having to become a statistic. It is extremely doubtful that answers and solutions will come from major breakthroughs in traditional medical science. Instead, we must focus our attention on the many actions and choices needing to be made in our daily lives that will steer us far away from the menacing world of breast cancer and the myriad health problems that threaten our children.

XX

When it comes to breast cancer, the experts tell us that it takes ten, fifteen or, perhaps, twenty years to develop. Therefore, the various contributing factors of this disease reach way back in time before anyone is even aware of the physiological storm that is brewing. Something has caused mal-adaptation of normal physiological processes, which has allowed the cells to go berserk.

So, if it takes a decade or more before breast cancer is detected and women in their 20's or 30's are now being diagnosed, then that means that the seeds of physiological disharmony are planted much earlier in time. Perhaps, even when they were fetuses floating in their mother's womb.

Could it be that hormone-disrupting chemical exposures in utero or during infancy set a time bomb ticking? What about nutrient deficient diets or the toxic foods our children eat daily? Could it be that the enthusiastic prescribing of oral contraceptives (which are made of two known carcinogenic drugs) to girls as young as 12 for conditions such as acne, PMS, irregular and painful periods and endometriosis are part of the problem?

Growing scientific evidence indicates so.

What Women MUST Know To Protect Their Daughters From Breast Cancer has a vital mission. It is to lift the veil of ignorance to reveal the many factors that presently jeopardize the hormonal health of our daughters.

Rather than feeling like helpless victims when it comes to protecting our children from breast cancer as well as halting other forms of hormone imbalances, there is, in fact, much that we can do.

The purpose of this book is to expose the underlying hormone disrupting influences that presently put our children at risk of hormonal imbalances and hormone dependent cancers.

The ensuing chapters will reveal the cancer culprits:

- Hormone disrupters in the environment and homes
- The role of estrogen mimics
- Synthetic hormones
- Pharmaceutical drugs
- Dietary indiscretions
- Underlying immune dysfunctions
- Nutritional deficiencies
- Cultural misperceptions

Once the veil has been lifted, we then must focus on finding solutions, creating the changes, initiating new behaviors, making new choices and weaving them all into our daily lives. *What Women MUST Know To Protect Their Daughters From Breast Cancer* is also an important resource providing many practical solutions and strategies for ensuring young women's hormonal health at all stages of their life - as fetuses, infants, children, adolescents, teenagers or young adults.

Although much of this book is focused on the challenges facing daughters, it's important to remember that your sons are also at risk of hormonal disruption and other serious health threats. There is an alarming increase in male genitalia deformities, low sperm counts and testicular cancers. In truth, we all live in a world, presenting all of us with many hurdles to maintaining lifelong good health.

This book is written to both warn and empower. It has vital information that parents and grandparents can use to safe guard the health of their children, grand children and future generations.

Teenagers and young adults will also benefit from what is found within these pages. They will learn to honor, respect and understand their bodies, and how return to hormonal balance, naturally.

The knowledge you gain and the informed choices you make now, this very moment, will chart a course for health – and establish a healthy foundation for life. The hormonal wellbeing of your children must be protected. Although the task is neither simple nor easy, it can be accomplished.

When fully armed with an understanding of the problem, proactive actions, and effective solutions, you can become an invincible force for change and good health. And with the knowledge you gain and the choices you make, you can insure your daughter's hormonal wellbeing and protect her from the growing risk of breast cancer.

There is much that needs to done. Your daughters are counting on you. So, let's begin.

PART ONE

Daughters at Risk!
What's Really Going On Here?

Something is definitely afoot in the breast cancer realm. Breast cancer is now creeping into the lives of younger and younger women.

It may come as a great surprise for many to learn the threat of breast cancer is now looming over 20 and 30 year old women. Hearing the words "you have breast cancer" is truly shocking at any age. But imagine what it's like when you're in the prime of your life.

While women in their thirties or younger, diagnosed with breast cancer may still be in the minority, the trend is increasing. **In fact, one in every 258 women between the ages of 30 and 40 will be diagnosed with breast cancer within the next ten years.**

These are the facts:

*Breast cancer is the leading cause of cancer death in young women ages 15–40.[1]

*Approximately 11,000 women under the age of 40 will be diagnosed with breast cancer this year, and close to 1,300 will die.[2]

*There are currently more than 250,000 women living in the United States under age 45 who have been diagnosed with breast cancer.

*Young women's cancers are generally more aggressive and less responsive to hormonal treatments and result in lower survival rates.

*The five-year relative survival rate for young women (those under 45 years of age) with breast cancer is 83 percent; this is slightly lower than the survival rate for women older than 45[3].

These are very sobering statistics.

Breast cancer will always be a tragedy that befalls a woman. It tears at the very fabric of a woman's life rippling out to touch all those in her world. The fears, uncertainties, and pain are deeply and profoundly shared by family, friends and co-workers. It is even a greater tragedy when young women are faced with this crisis because the tumors tend to be more aggressive. Young women also have to face the grim reality of a more advanced cancer at the time of diagnosis and higher mortality rates.

In addition, young women struggle with many other issues which don't concern their post-menopausal counterparts. Chemotherapy and radiation can initiate an early menopause. For some women this may temporarily shut down their ovaries. For others, however, the problem can be permanent resulting in infertility. Hot flashes, night sweats, insomnia and mood swings can be some of the on-going side effects. There is also the nagging uncertainty the cancer may one day return.

The following stories are the personal accounts of women whose lives were turned upside down when they suddenly found themselves fighting a life threatening disease. Needless to say, they were forever changed.

Not one of them ever suspected, at their age, they would be become a breast cancer statistic. A breast cancer diagnosis always comes as a shock; no one ever expects it, especially young, vibrant and seemingly healthy women. This was never supposed to happen; worse of all, young women are not suppose to die from this disease.

Here are five young women who were suddenly thrust into a life and death battle with the breast cancer monster.

Their stories were willingly told. They offer their lives as examples of how strength, courage and determination can overcome uncertainty and adversity. They also believe in being advocates. Knowing that when you have the courage to stand up for yourself, speak your mind, and tell people your own story changes happen. As they share their journeys, they know they have made a significant difference by inspiring other women to become more aware and to take better care of themselves. They also know their message is helping to save lives. These courageous women offer their stories as their most precious gifts of triumph and transformation.

Their stories are also a warning that lets everyone know the threat of breast cancer in young women is, indeed, real and much needs to be done stop this growing trend.

Jackie's Story

It was four days before Jackie's husband was to undergo heart surgery in March 2000. She was in the shower doing a routine breast self-exam. At first, she thought nothing of the marble sized lump. She thought to herself, "It's probably nothing, I'm young. Young women don't need to worry about breast cancer. I'll just keep a eye on it and see what happens." Besides, Jackie had more important things on her mind. Not wanting to concern her husband, she said nothing.

But only a week later, she noticed that the lump had grown even larger and was now painful. "I knew then, it wasn't something that was going to just go away. I had to see my doctor about it soon."

Her gynaecologist suggested she wait seven to ten days since the lump was most probably related to her menstrual cycle. She went back the next week concerned because the lump was growing larger and becoming more painful. He immediately sent her for a mammogram and sonogram, as well as referring her to a surgeon for a biopsy. Jackie had never experienced a mammogram. The x-ray machine was the largest piece of medical equipment she had ever seen. It took up the entire room. The technician placed her breast on the shelf. She cringed and clenched her fists. "I looked down at my breast. It was in the shape of a pancake, squished between two fiberglass plates.

After a few seconds, the pain was over.

A short time later, the head radiologist arrived and explained there was a suspicious area, 'a cluster of micro-calcifications.' The word cancer was not said at all. I thought that was a good sign, right? He was glad I had an appointment with a surgeon because they recommended I have a biopsy as soon as possible. They sent me on my way with a copy of the x-rays to take to my appointment. When I left, I was in a blur. I had no idea what they were talking about. Could this be bad? Could I have breast cancer?"

Five days later and a day before her 30th birthday, Jackie received the news she had dreaded. She had breast cancer. The biopsy showed that the cells were malignant. She listened to the report in total shock. Decisions had to be made and fast.

Two months later, Jackie had a lumpectomy. When she woke up from surgery, her husband told her the bad news. The cancer had spread. She was diagnosed with estrogen receptor positive invasive ductal carcinoma.

After healing from the surgery came the shock of chemotherapy, which she feared even more than surgery. It was advised to start treatment as soon as possible. She received chemotherapy every three weeks over a six-month period.

"The hardest part was losing my hair. It started falling out two weeks after I first started treatment. I also had lots of nausea but fortunately, I had drugs to control that. Chemotherapy put me into menopause right away. With that came the hot flashes. It was a bit hard to manage on top of being nauseous, feeling ugly and bald. It was really unpleasant. I just wanted to look normal so I wore a wig. However, my very pale skin and lack of eyebrows and eyelashes made that impossible. I was extremely self-conscious. I did go to work during all that time, except the day before and after chemotherapy. It was good for me because I would keep focused and busy. I tried to do my best to keep living every day as normally as I could."

Jackie finished chemotherapy in December. The doctor then dropped a ten-ton weight on her by announcing that he believed she had an 85 percent chance of developing the breast cancer in the other breast.

"When I was first diagnosed, I couldn't ever imagine losing a breast. But once I learned that the chances of developing breast cancer again were so high based on genetic information (I was a breast cancer gene carrier), I decided to have the mastectomy." Jackie had a double mastectomy with reconstruction. It was followed by 35 radiation treatments.

More than two years down the track, Jackie now takes a daily dose of the drug tamoxifen, which she will have to continue for the next five years. She still gets hot flashes. Three months after finishing chemotherapy, her menstrual cycles returned.

Jackie hopes to have a family, after finishing tamoxifen. "If I'm cancer free after five years we'll think about having a family at that time."

The chemotherapy has left its toll. Jackie can no longer be the runner she once was because the arthritis in her joints becomes too painful if she attempts to go for a jog. She now prefers walking.

Jackie doesn't really know what contributed to the genetic mutation. Was it primarily an inherited gene? Was it something in the environment? Was it the six years of taking the Pill? She has so many questions but no definitive answers.

"It doesn't really matter. What matters right now is getting on with life."

"Yes, I do worry about what the future holds for me, but now I know the importance of living each day to the fullest. Life holds new meaning for my husband and me. We've overcome so much in our short lives, and we've done it together. I tell him everyday that I couldn't get through even one day without him. He is my hero. He taught me how to be brave...

how to be strong. He says the same exact thing back to me! Our love for one another has grown more than I ever thought possible."

Rachel's Story

"You'll have to excuse me if I don't make much sense. I'm on quite a quantity of drugs," says 23 year old, Rachel, while reclining on the couch in her Auckland, New Zealand home. Rachel is referring to the cocktail of drugs that enters her system each week in a bid to fight metatastic disease - the advanced stage of breast cancer.

"I was 22 when I was diagnosed with breast cancer. I found the lump in my left breast myself and immediately went to my local GP, who, thankfully, took it very seriously. I had mammograms and an ultrasound. The next day I saw a breast surgeon who performed a core biopsy. Within a week from my first GP appointment I had been diagnosed with hormone receptor negative breast cancer. There is no history of breast cancer in my family and I had no other risk factors, so my diagnosis came as a big shock to my family and me. My tumor appeared quite large and the mammogram showed micro-calcifications, so it was decided that I would have a mastectomy."

In addition to a mastectomy, Rachel underwent breast reconstruction, had 4 different types of chemotherapies over 17 months of treatment, as well as 25 radiation treatments.

Rachel decided not to go back to work during her treatments. Instead, she planned to return to university and study for a Master's Degree in business management.

Everything was looking quite hopeful. Then one day while ironing, Rachel experienced back pain. She tried physiotherapy but it didn't appear to be helping. Rachel then decided to have a scan, which revealed a tiny broken bone in her vertebrae. She braced herself for the bad news. It was discovered her breast cancer had metastasized to her bones. All the many months of treatments had not halted the disease. Desperately trying to halt the disease, Rachel began using a powerful drug called Herceptin. Although not a cure, it has been known to put some people into remission for some time and allow them a good quality of life sometimes for months. Rachel also had three more single radiation sessions. In New Zealand, medical treatments and some medication are covered by their socialized medical system. In Rachel's case, the form of Herception she elected to take had not yet been approved for coverage by the government payment system, and the drug's cost was $10,000 per month. If she had to take another form of that drug, the side effects would have included lose of body hair, fingernails, toenails, horrendous nausea and a multitude of other horrible side effects.

"When you've been told you have a few months to live as I had, you don't want to be suffering with side-effects. You want to live," Rachel said.

After that, she had three good months and went back to university. But by then, the cancer had spread to her liver.

Rachel and her family had been attracting a great deal of media attention in New Zealand. Her father served in the Royal Air Force during the Vietnam War. At that time he was exposed to Agent Orange (dioxin). In other countries such exposure has been linked with spinal bifida, cleft palate and cancer in Vietnam veterans. Rachel's brother was born with a cleft palate. It was in everyone's mind, that Rachel's breast cancer might also be a legacy from her dad's exposure.

"Having breast cancer has made me realize we are fallible and can not protect ourselves from everything.

Some days I feel very angry and frustrated about what is happening but I can't change it, so I look to the positives. What I hold onto the most is I am aware of how precious life is and I try to make each day count."

Sadly, Rachel passed away a year and a half after first being diagnosed.

Penny's Story

At 26 years of age, Penny was on the fast track to a very successful career as a corporate communications consultant in New York City. It was a most stressful and demanding job that would often have her working 18-hour days or, unexpectedly, flying off to Europe at a moment's notice. It was an exciting life but an unpredictable one. For Penny, work came first and everything else came second, including her health. She would eat on the run, if she ate at all. Junk food was easy and convenient. "I truly believed that a fast food hamburger was a nutritious meal".

One evening while watching a television program about breast cancer, she decided to do her first breast self-exam. As her fingers explored her breasts, all seemed fine. However, she did feel some very strange small lumps right below her nipple. Not believing that it was anything to be alarmed about, she waited for 4 months before seeing a doctor.

She was in total shock when, sitting in her doctor's office, she was told that she had breast cancer. There must be a mistake. After all, 26-year-old women just don't get breast cancer. But indeed, the biopsy of the lump confirmed a tumor.

"I woke up one morning about a week after I found out I had breast cancer. I remember I was exhausted from hearing all of the options that the doctors wanted to try. They wanted to know what I wanted to try. So I outlined my choices. Number one: I could stay in bed and just die there. Number two: I could run away and die. Or, number three: I could get up and fight and hope for the best life possible during and after the fight."

"Of course I chose number three! I also picked the doctor of my choice and the operation of my choice, because it was my gamble and I truly was the one who would have to live with the results of my choice."

Penny decided to have a lumpectomy, which revealed positive margins. That means that the cancer could have already spread into the lymph system. The next step was to schedule 26 chemotherapy treatments. After that she agreed to a mastectomy. She chose not to do breast reconstruction.

"At first the scars were constant reminders of the bad things in my life...of the cancer...of the mastectomy...of my loss of innocence. And then one day they became true badges of courage and honor earned in a war that I fought to survive. The scars were the war wounds that proved I could survive even the toughest of battles."

"The mastectomy was one battle in that war. I made the strategic move to save my life. The scar that remains is my constant urgent reminder of how much I want to live, healthily and happily."

Although the cancer had not spread to her lymph nodes, Penny chose to take chemotherapy as a precaution against the cancer developing in other organs. She saw each chemotherapy treatment as another battle against her enemy. She knew the treatment would kill some of her healthy cells; but they were the unfortunate casualties of a fierce battle that was being waged inside her body.

When Penny reflects on the possible causes of her breast cancer, she immediately acknowledges the immense stress that had been her life. She also believes environmental exposure was a major contributor. It was easy for Penny to remember the terrible smell which would appear every Monday in her elementary school. "It was impossible to go to the bathroom because the smell of insecticide was so bad. I felt it would kill me. That horrible smell also permeated into the cafeteria. They must have sprayed the school with insecticide on Fridays."

Also, there was the experience when her mother was pregnant with her. Her mom had been complaining to the doctor of cramps and a lack of periods. When her pregnancy test came back negative, the doctor put her on a drug to induce a period.

She continued to use the drug (her mother couldn't remember what it was) for the next two months. A second opinion found the problem - pregnancy. Joy's mother worried throughout the entire pregnancy about the possible effects of that drug on her developing baby. However, her doctor reassured her that there was nothing to worry about. Penny was born a totally healthy looking baby. It was only 26 years later she once again questioned the possible effects of the drug taken during the first trimester of pregnancy. These are the questions that continue to haunt Penny.

Eight years later, Penny is a very different woman from that 26-year-old corporate whiz kid. She looks after herself much more vigilantly these days and pays keen attention to the needs of her body. She has become much more health conscious, eats a healthy diet and gets plenty of exercise. Penny is an avid white water kayaker. "Kayaking became a part of my heart and soul and motivated me to keep my arms strong." Penny is now married and has a beautiful seven-month-old baby boy. "If I was still that woman of 26, I would not be able to fully appreciate all I have now."

Ruth's Story

At 23 years old, Ruth, fresh out of college, moved to New York City to pursue her dreams. She always seemed to be a picture of health and vitality. One day, however, everything in her life suddenly changed.

"I found the lump in January. It was hard and smaller than a pea tucked away in my left breast, right under my armpit. I had gotten in the habit of doing a monthly self-exam while in college and kept it up since moving to New York City. I figured the lump was either a harmless cyst, like the one my mother had removed when she was my age, or nothing. At 23, it certainly couldn't be anything major. After my mother found out about the lump she wouldn't stop bugging me about it and reminding me that my dad's sister had breast cancer at age 31." Ruth tried to ignore it but the lump kept growing. She finally got a mammogram in June. The result was inconclusive, as it is for many young women whose breast tissue is relatively dense. She breathed a sigh of great relief. She was okay! The doctor said that young women like Ruth didn't fit the profile for breast cancer, but just to be on the safe side, he recommended an ultrasound. Ruth, however, tuned out his advice and decided to do it at a later date.

By November the lump was the size of a small marble. At her mother's constant urging, Ruth finally made an appointment to get an ultrasound. As she watched the doctor examine the images of her breast on the screen, she queried "It's a cyst, right?" The practitioner tonelessly replied, "No it wasn't." Then she said, "We'd better get a biopsy to see if it's malignant."

The doctor stuck a needle in the lump to collect sample cells. Ruth waited for about 10 excruciating minutes. As soon as she saw the doctor's face, her heart started pounding. "It's breast cancer," the doctor said softly. Ruth put her head in her hands and sobbed.

The very next day, almost one year after Ruth first discovered the lump, she had a lumpectomy. But the lumpectomy, which left a 2-inch scar under her armpit, was only the beginning. "The week after the lumpectomy was the worst week in my life. I waited to hear whether the cancer had spread; and what were my chances for survival. I was certain it had spread - I had let it go for a year. As other people were shopping for Christmas presents, I was imagining dying and how I was going to say good-bye to everyone. I also fantasized about trips I could take before I died."

Ruth got lucky. Her cancer had apparently not spread. It was stage 1 and estrogen receptor positive.

During the next few weeks, Ruth had to decide on a treatment plan. She assumed the doctors would simply tell her what was going to happen. Unfortunately, it wasn't that simple. Cancer treatment is far from being an exact science and the options vary. The doctors could only offer her different treatment alternatives and ultimately the decision was hers to make. She visited three different doctors hoping to arrive at a consensus. However, the only thing all the doctors agreed upon was she would have to undergo chemotherapy in order to treat what the doctors termed an aggressive, fast-growing cancer. They differed on the duration of the treatment and the specific medicines involved. One doctor recommended a prophylactic double mastectomy, but even that wouldn't guarantee that it wouldn't return.

After weighing all of her options, Ruth decided on four treatments of chemotherapy. These would be administered at three-week intervals. Additionally, she needed 7 weeks of radiation–ten minutes a day, five days a week to be followed by five years of tamoxifen.

"When I learned I had to undergo chemotherapy, I was petrified. I never knew anyone who had gone through chemo and really had no idea what it was, aside from the negative connotations that are always associated with it."

Ruth's a first chemo session was five hours long and she was hooked up to an IV that pumped powerful drugs into her blood stream. That night the nausea started, despite the preventative medication she was taking.

"Over the next few days, I was consistently nauseous. It was a pretty miserable time, but I knew it wouldn't last, and I just had to persevere through the worst of it."

Her second treatment, scheduled three weeks away, was delayed due to a low white blood cell count. "Despite the fact it was just a brief postponement, it was very frustrating. I think this was because I realized, despite the confidence of my doctors, I was completely at the mercy of my own body. No matter how positive an attitude I maintained, I could not simply will my body to be OK."

Three days later her cell count was high enough for treatment. "This time the nausea wasn't as intense, but it persisted for a couple of weeks. I didn't vomit, but instead suffered more of an upset stomach and flu-like symptoms. I also had hot flashes for a couple of days. After the second treatment, my doctors had me take shots to increase my white blood cell count. These shots have been the worst part of the whole ordeal to date. I administered them to myself at home. The drugs in those shots made my body so sore that I'd feel like I had worked out for ten hours straight"

A few days after the fourth treatment, Ruth caught a cold. Ordinarily, this would be no big deal but, with her weakened immune system, it really caused major discomfort. Instead of simply being an annoyance, it felt like a severe case of the flu. "My whole body ached, and I was horribly weak and dizzy. I couldn't even walk down the stairs without feeling like I was going to pass out. But besides this sickness, I felt a strange combination of relief and anxiety. I almost couldn't believe that I'd actually finished chemo and the worst of everything was behind me. But I couldn't escape the empty feeling that I could no longer rely on the drugs to keep the cancer away."

The radiation sessions were easier. She would whip her shirt off, lie down for ten minutes and then get her breast zapped, quickly and painlessly. However, the therapy made her feel exhausted.

"By the time my hair started to fall out, I was fully prepared for it. At that point, my scalp had started to ache, presumably from the hair loss. I decided it was time to shave it off completely.

"Once I accepted the fact that I was going to lose all of my hair, my biggest concern was over how others would react to my baldness. I didn't want my friends to feel uncomfortable seeing me without hair. I wanted to be sure that they knew that I was cool with it, and that they should be too. I needed them to feel as natural joking about my being bald as I did."

Ruth decided the easiest way to accomplish this was to involve her friends in the process. To do this, she threw a hair-cutting party. Letting all of her friends be involved in her process created greater support for Ruth. "They could openly talk to me about the cancer, and they've felt that way since."

Having the party was beneficial in other ways as well. It allowed Ruth to feel more in control of the situation, instead of at the mercy of chemo's side effects. It also allowed her to get adjusted to her hair loss.

"All along, I was secretly terrified that no matter how good I was, no matter how disciplined, no matter how hard I smiled, even if I felt like an aching, nauseous zombie, the cancer would come rushing back. The hospital arranged for me to join a support group of patients who were going through the same sort of hell. The support group helped a lot."

When Ruth finished her treatments she decided it was time to make some changes in her life. She quit her job and joined two rock groups to pursue her dream of being a musician.

"This experience taught me to live more in the moment. Everyday I try to do something new and to help educate other women about breast cancer."

After going through this ordeal, Ruth started dating a new guy. He made her promise never to grow her hair long again.

Lucy's Story

Lucy, a vibrant, talented and hard-working young Australian woman, bubbled over with an exuberance for life. Working in the entertainment world, her hours were demanding and so was her social life!

Lucy first noticed a lump in her breast when she was just

22 years old. "I thought I was much too young to get something like breast cancer, so I didn't really worry about it at all." Thinking it wasn't really anything to worry about, she chose to ignore it. However, two years later nothing had changed; she could still feel the lump in her breast. The thought of breast cancer never entered her mind. Although it hadn't grown any bigger, she decided to have her doctor check it out just to be on the safe side.

After six months of many doctor's consultations, Lucy finally learned the shocking news. Tests had conclusively shown that the lump was malignant. She was just 24 years old.

Her diagnosis was first thought to be an aggressive kind of cancer, but upon re-evaluation she was assured the prognosis was, in fact, very good. Even though the cancer hadn't spread at all, the decision was made to remove all of her lymph nodes. The rest of her treatment involved six weeks of radiotherapy.

"After the treatment, I went back to my crazy lifestyle and basically lived life the same way as before. I continued on my merry ol' way without any changes to my life. I totally believed my doctors when they told me to just carry on as normal. Don't change a thing. They told me that I had a really good prognosis, and chances were really slim that it will come back".

The one recommendation her doctor did advise was to immediately stop taking the pill, which she had been continuously using since the age of 15.

Reassured by her doctors, Lucy believed that she was out of the woods. She hadn't really given much thought to the whole breast cancer business. She was just glad that it was over and could carry on with life again. "I was complacent. It didn't really dawn on me what had happened and the second chance that I had been given."

Four years later, Lucy began to complain of back pains. During her doctor's appointment she was told the devastating news.

The cancer had returned. The pain she had been experiencing was due to the cancer that had now spread to her bones. "The first time I was diagnosed, I didn't know a thing about cancer. I guess I was in shock and just went along with whatever the medical profession said. It was all such a blur. I was numb throughout the whole experience. I didn't even cry until much later when I found out I was in the clear. It was all too hard to take in, so I guess my psyche dealt with it by numbing my feelings."

But now with this second diagnosis, the prognosis was worse–much worse.

"The specialist told me the cancer was going to get me; it was just a matter of time. It might be a broad stretch of time but it would get me in the end. The second time was different because I had to deal with it. Western medicine didn't offer me a lot of hope this time. I had to face it and really think about it. It was like some really bad dream that you wait to wake up from...and it just doesn't happen."

It was at this time Lucy experienced a profound change. It was as though both her inner resources and fighting spirit suddenly kicked in. "For whatever the reason I knew I would find a way. I never, ever felt it was hopeless even though I was told I didn't really have a chance."

Lucy decided to take charge of her therapy. She committed to a course of chemotherapy. However, she decided to have shorter course than what had been recommended so it wouldn't destroy all of her immune defenses afterwards. For the next twelve months, Lucy embarked upon a committed program using various forms of natural therapies, self-help techniques as well as some orthodox medicine. She focused on rebuilding her immune system. "I wholeheartedly believed my body could heal itself if given the right circumstances and tools to do so."

In the one year since she had been diagnosed with bone metastases, Lucy has made huge changes in her life. Instead of being a passive victim and accepting a rather hopeless situation, she decided to take charge of her healing and her life. In addition to incorporating holistic medicine into her program, she drastically changed her diet, eating predominantly organic foods and drinking pure water. As much as possible, she has cleaned up her toxic environment as well as her toxic thoughts.

Life looks most promising for Lucy these days. Recently, scans have shown that her bones are definitely healing. "I think in circumstances like mine, this is really unusual. You don't usually get better when cancer spreads to the bones. But in my case it's definitely getting better and improving. My bones are regenerating and healing."

"Actually getting out there and looking for the answers for myself, as well as making the effort to give the power back to myself, has made all the difference. This is where the majority of my healing has come from."

"Getting in touch with my spiritual side has been really important to me. Before all this happened, I didn't' think about the spiritual side at all. I was just too busy. It was all about living a very materialistic life. This has been a huge learning curve for me because I had to re-evaluate every aspect of my life. I am now a completely different person, and that's a good thing. I feel so much more balanced. Before, I was extremely out of imbalance which no doubt contributed to getting sick."

Lucy's experience with breast and bone cancer has been a profound transformative process. "This has been such a journey and I'm proud of myself for having the courage to have made so many changes. I'm so glad that I decided to take the path less traveled because it really has paid off."

Before we go much further in exploring the many causes putting our daughters at risk of breast cancer, we need to take a look at the gene factor. In an attempt to make sense of why this disease occurs, especially in young women, the culprit is usually preceived as an inherited mutant breast cancer gene. Most women are surprised to learn that the defective gene connection is present in only a very small percentage of women. In fact, according to the American Cancer Society, hereditary breast cancer makes up only 5 to 10 percent of all breast cancer cases.[1]

Genes, the building blocks of life's blueprint, have taken on almost magical powers. Medicine tells us that they are invisible forces that can pre-determine our future and hold the power to seal our fate.

When medical science lacks an accurate and comprehensive explanation for the cause of a disease process like breast cancer, then other theories are sought out. The medical community and the media, eager for a major breakthrough, greet these theories with great expectations. Since women and their medical doctors are really at a loss to explain the cause of breast cancer, the genetic mutation theory offered a plausible explanation.

In 1994 a breast-ovarian cancer susceptibility gene, known as BRCA1 (Breast Cancer-1) was discovered. This quickly led to the development of tests for the presence of other gene alterations potentially associated with breast cancer.[2] A second breast cancer susceptibility gene called BRCA2 and a third, BRCA3, have also been identified.

But, what are the real facts about breast cancer genes? The BRCA1 gene is actually present in everyone. When functioning normally, it is thought to suppress the growth of cancerous cells in the breast.[3] Metaphorically, it acts like a brake on a car. When altered, however, the gene permits runaway growth. This mutated gene results in uncontrolled cell growth increasing the risk for breast cancer or ovarian cancer.

According to Dr. Susan Love, renowned physician and best-selling author of *Dr. Susan Love's Breast Book*, "This risk factor is often exaggerated; Women come to me convinced that since their mother and aunt had breast cancer, they have a 50 percent chance of getting it. While it is true breast cancer in the family increases a woman's chance of getting breast cancer, the increased risk for most women may not be that great."[4]

Susceptibility Does Not Mean Inevitability

Shockingly, 70 percent of women with breast cancer have no known risk factors at all. Even if a woman were to be diagnosed with the BRCA gene, it is most important to understand susceptibility does not mean inevitability.

While mutated genes have a role in breast cancer, they are rarely the inherited kind. So, we must look elsewhere for other factors that compromise the DNA of a healthy cell. Dr. Janette Sherman, researcher and author of *Life's Delicate Balance: Causes and Prevention of Breast Cancer*, explains, "We know most babies arrive on this earth with fully functioning genetic systems, despite varying ethnic backgrounds. While some cancers may arise from an inherited genetic defect, we know many more arise from random damage to the genetic machinery of normal body cells. Genetic damage can also result from the formation of free radicals during normal metabolic processes. It is important to understand cancer develops in seemingly healthy people. We develop cancer when our bodies' normal functions, are altered by sub microscopic forces, chemical and physical."[5]

Far from an inherited condition that makes women feel like they are at the mercy of genes that have run amok, much of the cancer epidemic of today is a result of increasing exposure to chemical, radiation and pathogenic factors. Although most of us have susceptibility to one illness or another, a second triggering factor from the environment is needed to make the abnormality or disease manifest. Remember 90-95 percent of women do not have the breast cancer gene mutation.

Dr. Samuel Epstein, professor of occupational and environmental Medicine at the University of Illinois School of Public Health concurs. "Genetic factors obviously cannot account for the startling increases in breast cancer over the past decades. By concentrating on genetic research, then, the cancer establishment takes the hope of prevention out of the hands of most women. By far, the vast majority of breast cancer cases are linked to one or more environmental, medical or personal risk factors over which, you have far more control than you think."[6]

An Important Footnote to the Gene Theory

The gene theory in breast cancer has gained quite a foothold as an explanation for some types of breast cancer. Many healthy women who test positive for the gene will, out of sheer terror and ignorance, decide to have their breasts removed rather than live with the continual fear of an inevitable diagnosis.

However, serious questions have been raised about the relevance of the BRCA1 gene. For instance, what exactly are these gene mutations telling us? Are we looking at a cause or are we really looking at an effect?

The initial research of gene mutations was based on samples taken from Mormon families living in southwest Utah with a generational history of breast cancer. Mormon families are useful for genetic studies because they keep detailed, long-term genealogical records. Researchers from the University of Utah studied this particular population of women looking for the now famous BRCA1 gene.

By 1976, when the blood collection began, the Utah population had been subjected to gene damaging nuclear fallout from the Nevada test site for the past 25 years. A total of 26 above ground nuclear tests and 11 underground tests had been detonated between 1951 and 1980. When the bomb testing was finally stopped, there was an excess incidence of cancer (61 percent for all ages) in Mormon families who lived in southwestern Utah and adjacent areas of Nevada and Arizona. By 1996, when the blood collection was completed for the gene identification study, 45 years of radiation exposure had passed. That's more than enough time for radiation exposure to have caused significant genetic damage.[7]

Considering the cancer clusters and the BRCA1 gene were first identified in Utah, could the genetic alterations actually have been caused by the radioactivity carried from the Nevada test site contaminating the homes and farms of these families?

Additionally, there is no way of knowing if the defective BRCA1 gene had, in fact, been an inherent defect. Could the Utah "clan of one-breasted women", as these Mormon women were called, have suffered genetic damage from the radiation exposure they had been exposed to from past decades of nuclear testing? In addition to radiation, what other gene-damaging stimuli were active? What about other insults from many years of pesticide exposure? Perhaps other hormone-disrupting chemicals had tainted their food, fish and livestock?

Far from finding a missing piece to the breast cancer puzzle, more uncertainty has been created. More questions are in search of answers. What part did each or all of these events play in altering the breast cancer gene? When, in the course of time, did these genetic variations first appear? Since these questions remain undetermined and unanswered, the real meaning of the BRCA genes is still far from certain.

It appears that too much emphasis has been placed on breast cancer genes as the cause for the growing incidence of breast cancer in all women. Metaphorically, genes may load the gun, but what really pulls the trigger?

If genes aren't the definitive answer, the underlying causes of breast cancer must be found elsewhere.

"We should always be humbled when we think of what we do not know about the female reproductive cycle. We still have no understanding of the mechanism that makes one Graafian follicle in one ovary of a normal woman maturate and ovulate each month. This is a baffling problem. Until we know the mechanism that selects one Graafian follicle, out of perhaps hundreds of thousands, to maturate each month, we still have to proceed with caution on any long-term hormonal treatment of the human female."

These cautionary words were the warning given by Sir Charles Dodd, the English chemist who developed the first synthetic estrogen called DES (diethylstilbestrol) in the 1930's. It was non-patentable, very cheap and was about to open a Pandora's box of misery.

Since laboratory experiments showed DES to be a very potent estrogen, Dodd intended DES to be used only for the short term and only for conditions of estrogen deficiency. In fact, from the very start studies showed mice exposed in utero to DES developed breast cancer, malformed reproductive organs and liver cancer.

As early as the 1930's, other studies showed tinkering with hormone levels during pregnancy was dangerous business, particularly for the fetus undergoing rapid development in the womb. By 1938, Sir Charles Dodd was also sure of one other thing. The synthetic estrogen, DES, could cause breast cancer.

Disregarding these ominous warnings, the FDA approved DES in 1947 as a drug to prevent miscarriage.

Prescribing A Lie

Despite no controlled studies had been conducted to determine the effectiveness or safety of DES for use during pregnancy, drug companies promoted this drug with all the gusto they could muster. Before long, DES was being prescribed to women not only to prevent miscarriage, but also as a wonder drug to "make a normal pregnancy more normal", to stop lactation, for menopausal symptoms, for acne and as a morning after pill.

Farmers were equally bullish on DES and used tons of it as an additive to animal feed or implanted it in neck or ear as a growth promoter in chickens, cows, pigs and other livestock.

For more than thirty years, this enthusiastic yet unproven prescribing of DES was given to more than ten million American women and many more millions of women worldwide.

The DES Debacle

By 1953 it was well established DES did not prevent miscarriage. In fact, studies showed DES actually increased the rate of miscarriage. However, it wasn't until 1971 the FDA finally issued an alert advising against the use of DES during pregnancy. Even though DES was a hazard to pregnant women, it was never banned from human use or taken off the market. It is still in use as an anti-miscarriage drug in many developing countries such as China and Mexico.

In 1971 Dodd's dire warnings came true. A rare form of an aggressive and lethal form of vaginal cancer was showing up in a growing number of young women whose mothers used DES. The "wonder drug" now emerged as the "Frankenstein drug".

Although the children born to DES mothers looked perfectly normal at birth, the hormone disrupting effects from DES use in utero finally came to light. DES caused cancer, especially estrogen sensitive cancers, and it crossed the placental barrier causing reproductive abnormalities in both females and males. Deformed uteruses, infertility, predispositions to reproductive problems, such as heavy and painful periods, endometriosis, ovarian cysts, fibrocystic breast disease, and compromised immune systems have now been found in daughters born to

DES mothers. These women were also more predisposed to breast cancer.

In males, smaller penises and other genital abnormalities, a greater incidence of testicular cancer, and compromised immunity were part of the DES legacy. The mothers who took DES were also affected. Many were developing breast cancer. There is further evidence suggesting the chromosomal damage from DES will be passed onto the third generation.

The unrestrained prescribing of DES has now been written into the annals of women's history as a disastrous medical experiment conducted on trusting women and their unborn children. It was not the first medical disaster that caused untold pain and suffering and, unfortunately, will most certainly not be the last.

The important lessons gleaned from the thirty years of DES exposure impacts profoundly on all of us at this time. The use of the first synthetic estrogen revealed prolonged and pervasive hormone disrupting effects on the women who took the drug but casts a dubious shadow on the hormonal health of their offspring.

Until DES, most scientists believed a drug was safe unless it caused immediate and obvious malformations. The DES debacle revealed drugs could create long-term impact without causing any outwardly visible birth defects. The hormone disasters were only discovered years down the track.

Charles Dodd' pioneering work also found chemicals appearing like estrogens, even ones that didn't, could act like estrogens. He was the first to recognize estrogen-like activity in chemical compounds. This included not only DES but also many other commons chemicals found in plastics and detergents.

The era of synthetic hormones and hormone disrupting drugs and chemicals had begun.

There is a direct connection between estrogen and breast cancer. For more than 100 years, estrogen's intimate relationship to breast cancer has been observed.

Hormones are chemical messengers produced in one area of the body and transported in the blood to act at another place of the body, such as cells or organs. Hormones are released from the brain, thyroid, ovaries, testes and other endocrine glands and then carried through the bloodstream to the target cells and organs where they activate and regulate various functions.

Natural hormones, those made in the body, live rather short lives, staying in the blood stream for only a few minutes or at most a few hours - just long enough to do their jobs. They don't accumulate in the tissues and are easily broken down and eliminated from the body. The same cannot be said about synthetic hormones or hormone-disrupting chemicals. Synthetic hormones, found in birth control pills and hormone replacement therapy, remain longer in the body than natural hormones. However, pesticides and other environmental compounds last much longer.

What natural hormones lack in the time they are active, they make up in their potency. As powerful messenger molecules, which create very dramatic changes in cell activity, hormones are released in minute amounts - parts per billion or even parts per trillion. Estrogens, for instance, are measured in parts per trillion. To get a sense of what parts per billion is like imagine placing one drop of water into a six-mile-long train with 660 tank cars! This very teeny tiny amount will initiate a very powerful physiological response.

Estrogen, made primarily in the ovaries, is the class of hormones most responsible for programming the way the body grows. Estrogen exposure in the womb is also necessary to program the developing fetus to respond to other hormones later in life.

Natural estrogens have important work to do. They cause

specific cells to enlarge and divide. In addition, they control reproductive cycles and pregnancy; prepare the breasts for lactation, influence the skin, the bones and the cardiovascular system, the immune system and even the brain.

When estrogen levels are in proper balance the body hums along supporting life's processes. However, when estrogen is in excess, it takes on a more sinister role, and wreaks havoc in the body. One of estrogen's jobs is to proliferate cell growth. It's the hormone that causes secondary sex characteristics in females, such as, breast development and curvy hips. Its message to estrogen sensitive cells is to grow, grow, and grow. When estrogen is excessive, out-of-control growth contributes to various problems, including breast, uterine and ovarian cancers.

The evidence is overwhelming; excess estrogen is intimately connected to the development of the majority of breast cancers. Estrogen encourages breast cells to divide more often and more rapidly. If a mutation (either inherited or triggered by a carcinogen) lies embedded in the DNA, cancer cells are more likely to proliferate when high estrogen levels are present.

Two distinct types of breast cancer exist. The far more common estrogen-dependent breast cancer, or estrogen receptors positive, is influenced primarily by estrogen. The less common form is non-estrogen-dependent, also known as estrogen negative. More than two-thirds of women with breast cancer have estrogen dependent cancer.

When the endocrine system is working properly, it communicates its messages by secreting a hormone that travels through the bloodstream and delivers its communication to a special protein called a receptor. A receptor looks like an open pouch. It acts very much like a lock that is opened by a hormonal key. When a hormone enters the binding site, it fits neatly into the pouch and the hormone is bound to the receptor.

Receptors are located either on the surface of cells, or in the cell's nucleus. They act like an on-off switch for a particular activity in the cell. If the right substance comes along that fits the receptors the switch is turned on and a particular activity in the cells begins. Estrogen is a very important "key" for the many receptor sites found on cells throughout the body.

Estrogen travels through the blood stream and finds its matching receptor sites on both healthy cells and cancer cells. Once the estrogen fits into the receptor, the switch is turned on. It then sends a strong signal to the nucleus, the 'headquarters' of the cell. The message is unmistakable: Grow, create new cells and keep growing.

Hormone disrupting compounds are great mimics. Like saboteurs, they can mimic certain hormones, such as estrogen, slipping into receptor sites and create inappropriate messages – turning some processes on, some off or blocking messages altogether.

Estrogen receptor positive breast cancer cells can grow only if they are "fed" by excess estrogen or estrogen-like chemicals.

Why is estrogen-dependent breast cancer so much more common today than it was just a few decades ago? It has become much more obvious women around the world are now exposed to more estrogen and for a longer time than ever before. Signs of this estrogen excess are even appearing in children. Young girls are going into puberty at much earlier ages. Estrogen must be present in sufficient amounts to trigger this kind of unnatural change.

When examining the reasons for the growing number of estrogen initiated breast cancers, we need to explore the many ways that excessive amounts of estrogen have entered not only our world but also our bodies.

Continuous exposure to various forms of estrogens and estrogen-like chemicals throughout one's life, from the moment of conception, through childhood, adolescence and into adulthood, is signalling and activating powerful hormonal messages. The consequences of these aberrant communications to the receptor sites pave the way for estrogen dependent cancers, especially breast cancer.

One source of estrogen exposure comes from the introduction of synthetic estrogens found in birth control pills and hormone replacement therapy. The pharmaceutical industries have developed a wide variety of synthetic estrogens. These kinds of estrogens are more powerful, more potentially carcinogenic and longer lasting in the body than are the natural estrogens. In some cases they can be hundreds of times more potent than naturally made estrogens.

Like pouring fuel on a fire, prolonged exposure to any kind of estrogen significantly increases the risk for developing breast cancer, especially estrogen receptor positive cancer.

But, by far, the most dangerous estrogens are found not in our bodies, but in the chemicals released into the environment.

Throughout the history of humanity, hormonal signals have always come from inside our bodies or from natural substances, such as estrogen plants, that have evolved along with us. Since World War II, something unprecedented has occurred. Millions of man-made chemicals used in the external world have been entering the environment. We have now discovered many of these chemicals act as hormones. Unfortunately, from an evolutionary point of view, our bodies have not had enough time to protect us from these alien messengers. No organism on earth has evolved to deal with these human produced chemicals.

We presently live in a world that is inundated with tens of thousands of different chemicals that are now known to have hormonal actions. These diverse chemicals are known as hormone disruptors. Very little study has been done on their long-term safety or their combined effects on living organisms. However, the emerging evidence of their consequences is most evident.

Drowning in a Sea of Hormone Disrupters

Hormone disruptors, also known as endocrine disruptors, are specific chemicals or mixtures of chemicals from outside the body that can disrupt the development or function of the hormonal systems leading to irreversible adverse health effects.

These synthetic chemicals find their way into our bodies through the food we eat, the water we drink and bathe in and the air we breathe.

Thank goodness for the wildlife biologists. Dedication to their science has alerted us to important and alarming changes happening to our world - changes that are presently occurring everywhere. They have been crucial in helping us to recognize and understand the hormonal effects of environmental contaminants.

Scientists studying wildlife all across the globe have reported ominous findings of disease, mutations and death linked to environmental pollution. In some cases, entire species have suddenly and mysteriously disappeared. Exposure to toxic chemicals, possessing unintended hormonal actions, has resulted in anatomic, physiologic, reproductive, carcinogenic and behavioral abnormalities to all forms of animal life. Amphibians, fish, reptiles and mammals are all suffering the effects of global contamination.

These widespread adverse effects have been attributed to the hormone disruptors gaining entrance to the bodies of animals and humans alike. They weaken defenses and wreak their havoc of cancer, hormonal disruption, immunological abnormalities and birth defects.

Our world is now awash in endocrine disrupting chemicals; chemicals that biologically alter the hormonal nature of all animal life. They are found everywhere on earth, from the most remote arctic wilderness to the greatest depths of the ocean.

Warnings from Nature

Lake Mead is one of the most popular vacation spots in the United States and a main source of drinking water for Southern California and Las Vegas, Nevada. Treated and untreated waste, including chemical waste and pesticides, has been dumped directly into the lake for many years.

Indisputable signs of something going terribly wrong have started to appear. Funny things are happening to the fish. Male carp are making egg protein usually produced only by females, making them hermaphrodites, exhibiting both male and female characteristics.

This phenomenon is not solely restricted to the United States. It's occurring worldwide. In England and Australia, fish exposed to estrogenic compounds from liquid sewage waste released into their rivers are also changing sex. This waste is released into half of the water that flows into English rivers during the summer where more than 30% of it becomes drinking water.

Upon closer scrutiny, a shocking discovery was made. The feminization of the male fish had been caused by sewage contamination from the estrogens in women's urine who were using synthetic hormones. Millions of women using hormone replacement therapy and oral contraceptives were unknowingly causing this contamination. Since the estrogens and progestins found in HRT and all forms of hormone contraceptives are known carcinogens, as well as hormone contaminants, the long term consequences of this type of exposure is just beginning to be assessed.

Japanese researchers have also discovered similar feminization of three fish species living in marine waters around Japan. This surprised the scientists since they expected the dilution effect of marine waters to be sufficient to negate any inputs of endocrine disrupting compounds. Three species are involved which indicates this is a widespread phenomena. The research indicates "the prevalence of the feminized fish is greater in waters near urban areas producing large amounts of industrial and household waste water."[1]

If the fish are being so profoundly altered by their exposure to these hormone disruptors, just what might be happening to all the people who are not only swimming in the lake but also drinking the water?

If that discovery wasn't chilling enough, scientists discovered when DDT was injected into male fish, they changed into the opposite sex capable of laying eggs and producing baby fish. The study also confirmed the DDT contaminated fish could pass their toxins through their eggs, profoundly altering development of the next generation. Although the US banned DDT decades ago, it persists for decades and is still used in some developing countries.

Organochlorines are chlorine-based chemicals. They are also extremely toxic and lethal. They include herbicides, pesticides, including DDT, its metabolite DDE, dieldrin, atrazine, methoxychlor, hetachlor, kepone, chlorine beach, most disinfectants, various plastics and vinyl chloride found in plastic products like baby bottles and baby's soft toys.

Over 90 percent of the population applies 300 million pounds of these poisons annually, often indoors. Surprisingly, city dwellers use more chemicals per acre than farmers. In a lifetime, 50 pounds of toxic waste can enter a body from drinking water and at least 450 pounds can enter the body through the skin. They accumulate in the body in many ways: from drinking water, food grown with agricultural chemicals, plastic migrating into canned and microwaved foods, and food or body contact with chlorine bleached paper products (coffee filters, tampons, paper cups, toilet papers).

Although pesticides are designed to kill insects and other pests, that's not all they do. In fact, only 2 percent of the 1.2 billion pounds of pesticides sprayed on crops annually accomplish this purpose! The other 98 percent are absorbed into the air, water, soil, or food supply and into our bodies.

The majority of organochlorines are stored in fat cells and breast tissue. Some are eliminated in tears, breast milk and egg cells or sperm. The tendency for organochlorines to stay in the body is evidenced by the recent samples of fat and breast milk collected from women in the United States and Canada contained DDT, chlordane and dieldrin. These organochlorines have been banned for over three decades.

Women with high levels of agricultural organochlorines in their blood are 4 to 10 times more likely to develop breast cancer than women with low levels.

Women with breast cancer have 50-60 percent more PCBs, DDE and other pesticides and organochlorines in their tissues than women without breast cancer. For each 10–part per billion (ppb) increase in tissue levels of PCBs and DDE there is a 1 percent increase in breast cancer. Women in the United States and Canada currently have 300ppb PCBs and 1000 ppb DDE in their breast tissues. These two organochlorines alone could cause the 1-2 percent yearly increase in breast cancer seen in industrialized nations each year for the past 50 years.[1]

Gender bending is happening before our very eyes. No species is immune. Not even our own. What was once considered animal anomalies have now coalesced into a discernible pattern. Our worldwide environment and everything living is permeated by chemicals found in pesticides, herbicides, insecticides, organochlorine chemicals found in plastics, diesel exhaust, shampoos; steroid hormones found in oral contraceptives and hormone replacement therapy and the 87,000 chemicals presently in commercial use. They are also changing and damaging our bodies and creating a chain reaction jeopardizing the health of future generations.

This contamination is now known to alter animal's physiology in a number of ways. For example, wildlife researchers found birds exposed to xeno-estrogens show reproductive failure, growth retardation, life-threatening deformities and alterations to their brains and liver function.[1]

It wasn't only animal physiology that is changing; it is also their sexual behavior. For instance, female seagulls are nesting with other female seagulls.

In some animals sexual deformities are more common; female polar bears grew penis-like stumps; panthers have atrophied testicles. Fertility is also declining. In one alligator species from a contaminated Florida lake, 75 percent of the alligator eggs in the lake were dead or infertile. Turtles from the same lake also showed intersex conditions - a combination of male and female sexual characteristics.

It has now become apparent that no ecosystem has been left untouched. No human has been born since the middle of the 20th century without some exposure in the womb to hormonally active compounds.[2] Each new baby coming into this world already has as many as 500 foreign chemicals in its body.

Some of the synthetic chemical compounds are notorious because they accumulate in fatty tissue. These chemicals can then bioaccumulate up the food chain, and can be passed on in the womb and through breast milk. Because they are not flushed through our bodies, chemical accumulation in the fat tissue and breast milk can reach very high concentrations over time.

Chapter 10
Hormone Havoc

As scientific research on endocrine disruption has advanced, the scope of the research has broadened significantly. The list of hormonally active compounds is longer than anyone had previously imagined in the early days of the research. Not only are more compounds involved, but also more hormonal systems are now known to be vulnerable. Within each hormonal system, new mechanisms of interaction between compounds and receptor systems are being explored to understand how a compound exerts its effects.

But hormone disruption is not limited to estrogenic compounds or the estrogen receptors. To begin with, scientists have learned that there is more than one estrogen receptor, Further more, the mechanisms of disruption are diverse and complex; a compound may be an agonist (mimicking the actions of a hormone) or antagonist (interfering or blocking actions of a hormone); it may alter transport of a hormone; or it may bind to more than one hormone receptor.

Because every hormone system is potentially vulnerable to disruption or alteration, the list of hormone systems investigated has broadened beyond the sex hormones. While the first two decades of research focused largely on man-made chemicals capable of mimicking estrogen, within the past five years research has expanded to include estrogen blockers, androgen (male hormone) blockers, progesterone blockers and compounds that interfere with the thyroid. This last one is especially important because the thyroid hormone is key to proper brain development.

This means the sea of hormonally active chemicals, in which the fetus develops, may forever change the health and function of adults, and in some cases, may alter the course of an entire species. Worldwide, there are reports of declining sperm counts and a reduced ratio in births of male babies. Without the capacity to reproduce, a species ceases to exist. Extinction is forever; a species loss has never been reversed.

The data derived from animal observations are unequivocal; breast and genital cancers, genital abnormalities, interferences with sexual development and changes in reproductive behavior are all expressions of a root cause.

It now turns out many more systems are altered in addition to the endocrine system. Natural chemical signals are important at all levels of organization of life—within cells, among cells, between organs, even between organisms, including from one species to another. Any of these chemical signals, in principle, are vulnerable to disruption. Scientists have just begun to look at the chemical signals that mediate communication between symbiotic organisms, such as, nitrogen-fixing bacteria and the roots of the plants in which they live. They are examining how synthetic chemicals might interfere with these signals. Disrupting these 'signals of life' could have important ecosystem impacts.

The world we now live in poses threats to all of humanity never before known. Our children are the most vulnerable inhabitants of such a toxic hormonally disrupted world. Dianne Dumanoski, one of the authors of *Our Stolen Future*, sums up the challenge before us. "The next century stretches ahead of us like an urgent question. The problem isn't simply we don't have the answer. Our actions suggest the leaders of our now global civilization don't fully grasp the dilemma confronting us. We might get a better fix on our dilemma and target our efforts more effectively if we understood this as a 'humanity crisis' rather than an environmental crisis. Whatever else is in jeopardy, this is first and foremost a crisis for humans and our current civilization. By now it should be clear that we must stop chasing brush fires and take on the pyromaniac." [1]

The contamination is now very widespread and it comes from many sources, some quite conspicuous and others completely unexpected. Since we can't escape it, we must learn to take the precautions necessary to minimize our exposure. We can create our own safe havens while we actively demand greater environmental changes. The daily choices we make; about what we eat, the purity of the water we drink, what we spray on our lawns and the cleaning products we use in out home, all make a difference to the healthy development of our children and ourselves. Creating and maintaining healthy bodies, healthy homes, and healthy environments are imperative.

Like canaries in the proverbial coal mine, women with breast cancer, especially young women, are providing a dire warning of the silent invaders sabotaging our hormonal systems. It's time to lift the blinders and see what is really going on. Breast cancer is really not such a mystery. The real mystery is why so little is being done to make the changes.

Health Consequences

Hormone Disrupting Compounds

Pesticides – chemicals which include herbicides, fungicides and insecticides used on food crops, home gardens, flea collars, lice shampoo etc.

Plastics – both in their manufacture and disposal. Certain plastics when burned in incinerators can release dioxins, potent hormone disrupters.

Phthalates – compounds added to some plastics to make them more flexible and are able to migrate into whatever substance is being stored. They are used in polyvinyl chloride (PVC). They are found in synthetic leathers, adhesives, caulking, nail polish, deodorant, hair spray, perfumes, infants soft plastic toys they are also used as a component of paper and paperboard that comes in contact with liquid, fatty and dry foods.

Pharmaceuticals – birth control pills, hormone replacement therapy, fertility drugs, estrogen implants used in cattle.

Persistent Organic Pollutants – Made from chlorinated or brominated chemicals, which make substances more stable and more persistent. Pops are also ingredients in pesticides.

Health Consequences

From Hormone Disuptors

•Increased risk for indirect and/or ireversible genetic damage, laying the ground work for cancers later in life.

•Reproductive risk for menstrual irregularities, fallopian tube malfunctions, cervical and uterine defects; increased risk of endometriosis, cysts and fibroids.

•Increased risk of abnormal cell changes on the cervix and vagina.

•More autoimmune problems such as lupus, arthritis, diabetes, asthma and chronic respiratory infections.

•Women may be more prone to breast and ovarian cancer due to exposure in the womb and during youth when breast cells are most immature and more prone to damaging signals.

Hormone Disrupting Compounds

Polychlorinated biphenyls (PCBs) – had been used in transformers and other electrical equipment.

Dioxins – by products of chemical processes involving chlorine and released into the environment.

PVC (polyvinyl chloride) - most common of plastics and often mixed with phthalates, Manufacture of PVC and burning of PVC plastic generate large quantities of dioxins.

Detergents (alkylphenol ethoxylates, APEs) – class of chemical surfactants that dissolve and remove oils and grease and makes products more water-soluble. Found in commercial detergents, hair dyes, shampoos, shaving gels, cosmetics, spermicides, latex paints, industrial detergents for degreasing engine parts.

Heavy Metals – lead, cadmium and mercury. Found in lead crystal, plumbing, PVC, batteries, old paint tin cans; NiCad batteries, stabilizers

Environmental Hormone Disruptor Facts

Hormone Disrupting Compounds

• Every year, manufacturers around the world produce an estimated billion pounds of phthalates, the softeners used in vinyl and solvents used in cosmetics which are known to be hormone disruptors.

• The U.S. Centers for Disease Control and Prevention recently found a chemical found in nail polish, perfumes, mosquito repellents, some adhesives and some inks called dibutyl phthalate. DBP is known to interfere with hormones.

• Children 6 months to 4 years old have the highest daily exposure to the hormone-disrupting plastic softener used in vinyl (PVC), called di (2-ethylhexyl) phthalate (DEHP), from combined sources, such as foods, indoor air and water. National Toxicology Program, U.S. Dept. of Health and Human Services.

• From 1987 to 1993, over 500,000 pounds of the hormone-disrupting plastic softener used in vinyl (PVC), called di (2-ethylhexyl) phthalate (DEHP), were released into land and water in the U.S., according to EPA's Toxic Chemical Release Inventory. U.S. Environmental Protection Agency, Office of Water.

Environmental Hormone Disruptor Facts

• The rate of cancer among American children younger than fifteen has been steadily rising at a rate of nearly 1 percent per year over the past twenty years.

• Indoor levels of pollutants may be 2 to 5 times, and occasionally more than 1,000 times, higher than outdoor levels

• Parabens, which may interfere with hormones, are the most widely used cosmetic preservatives in the U.S.

• Bisphenol-A, which is used to make polycarbonate plastic - and a chemical that interferes with hormones - is one of the top 50 chemicals produced in the U.S. Over 1.6 billion pounds were produced in 1995.

• On average, humans ingest approximately 6.3 micrograms per day of bisphenol-A, the building block of polycarbonate plastic from the linings of food cans.

• U.S. production and use of hormone-disrupting alkylphenol ethoxylates (APEs), used in laundry detergents and shampoos, exceeded 450 million pounds in 1990

• Every year, manufacturers around the world produce an estimated billion pounds of phthalates, the softeners used in vinyl and solvents used in cosmetics which are known to be hormone disruptors.

PART TWO

What's Happening To Our Baby Girls?

Chapter 1
Babies At Risk

We usually think of life in the watery womb experience as a blissful time. Held within a protected bubble, the fetus floats in it own universe, growing and developing along the evolutionary pathway to humanhood. We think of the womb as a haven, an impermeable, all-protecting nirvana that shields new life from the dangers existing in a more tumultuous and toxic outside world. At least, for a time, the developing child is perfectly safe.

The protective placenta is a truly amazing organ. It surrounds the fetus and attaches to the mother, controlling metabolic changes. By month three of pregnancy, a human placenta is two inches in diameter. The attached umbilical cord is about four inches long. It will eventually grow into a curly twenty-two-inch-long, half inch wide rope. The placenta will expand into a disc that is eight inches wide and an inch thick that weighs slightly more than a pound. The placenta is expelled with the fetus during birth.

The placental barrier consists of a four-layer, semi-permeable membrane separating maternal and fetal circulation. When we say something crosses the placenta, we mean it passes through this membrane. Inside the placenta are capillary-filled branches soaked by spumes of mother's blood. The placental barrier does an admirable job of keeping out bacteria which are usually too large to pass into the placental branches. Those that do manage to sneak by are swiftly dispatched by special immune agents.

However, in recent years scientists have had to revise their perception of an impenetrable placental fortress. When it comes to toxic chemicals, the placenta is not really a barrier at all. Chemicals substances that are carried in the mother's circulation are sorted by the placenta primarily on the basis of molecular weight, electrical charge and fat solubility. In other words, molecules that readily dissolve in fat are afforded free passage regardless of their capacity for harm. In a sense it's a totally free ride for many toxins!

Unrestricted Entrance

As a lifelong advocate for women's health, scholar and author D. Lindsey Berkson has been investigating the effects of hormone disruptors on the fetus. In her book, *Hormone Deception*, she warns of the many dangers a developing fetus confronts within the womb.

> "During critical times such as pregnancy, a mother's body has high levels of estrogen. Fortunately 99 percent of the estrogen a pregnant woman makes is attached to sex hormone-binding globulin (SHBG). When estrogen rides piggyback on these blood proteins, it is said to be bound. Estrogen that is bound does not cross the placental barrier, so the estrogen cannot enter the body and brain of the developing child. The estrogen that is not bound is referred to as free estrogen as it is able to pass freely into cells and bind with receptors. Free estrogen is thus the biologically active estrogen that can get into a cell and send a signal to start estrogenic activity. Only 0.2 or 0.3 percent of a mother's estrogen is free and can get into the fetus.
> At this time it is thought that most xeno-estrogens do not bind with these blood proteins. DES is not bound at all with the sex hormone binding proteins in the blood. Xenoestrogens, therefore, circulate freely and have access to places where natural estrogens cannot tread. Even if these chemicals are much weaker than natural estrogens outside the body, their

potency increases inside the body because of their unrestricted travel capabilities.

Environmental estrogens can travel across the placenta and enter the growing fetus. These estrogens can be stored in the placenta, which has a large fat content, and slowly releases toxins to the developing fetus. Although these substances might not be nearly as potent as natural hormones when they are tested outside the body, xenoestrogens are more potent within the body than testing would suggest - parts per trillion can have an influence. When a compound like DES is introduced into the body and doesn't bind with the blood proteins, it can be as much as 100 times more potent than natural estradiol in the fetus. In another example, bisphenol A, by not binding to SHBG, has higher activity levels in the fetus than when tested in the lab.

Fetal exposure to hormones can program the way genes function for the rest of a person's life. Some gene's are suppose to get turned on early in life, some later. If a fetus or developing child is exposed to a potent hormone disruptor during a specific window of vulnerability, the path their cells take in his or her development may be altered, possibly permanently. A girl may show signs of puberty at age five instead of during early teen years. A boy's testicles may not descend. Intelligence may be affected. Sustained attention or response to stress may be altered. Individuals respond differently to these different signals."[1]

No Safe Haven

Consider pesticides. Those with low molecular weight

cross the barrier without restrictions. For them, it is like a free toll road. Pesticides made of bigger, heavier molecules are partly metabolized by the placenta's enzyme before they pass through, but sometimes this transformation turns into a more toxic chemical. The fetus is then placed at even greater risk. These days, the amniotic fluid, in which the unborn baby floats in for nine months most likely contains several pesticides. One study showed one third of the unborn babies floated in intrauterine fluid containing DDT, lindane and PCBs. DDT can interfere with the reproductive system's biochemical pathways; PCBs have been linked to birth defects and problems with the thyroid contributing to changes in both the nervous and immune systems

It is now known that DDE levels, a metabolite of DDT, is in the umbilical cord blood of newborn infants and are about one-third the DDE level in the mother's blood at the time of birth. A Japanese study released in April 1999 showed even higher levels. Researchers found the umbilical cord blood (as well as placenta and breast milk) had about 90 percent of the DDE level found in the mother's blood stream.[2]

Once the pollutants are shuttled cross the placenta, the fetus has far fewer resources for getting rid of toxins than does the mother. While in the womb, a fetus cannot transform chemicals very well at all. The unborn baby lacks a fully functioning liver and kidneys which can clear out pollutants. These chemicals take a one-way ride. When they get inside the womb, most of them take up permanent residence. This is one primary reason the fetus is extremely sensitive to all sorts of environmental insults.

The fetus may build up toxins from the mother's circulation even if the mother is successfully clearing herself. The fetus is exceptionally sensitive to contaminants crossing the placenta and even more so during the time its organs are being formed.

These hormonal disruptors are so powerful, that just one harmful dose during a woman's pregnancy can cause harmful effects
to her child many years down the road.

For instance, the higher the level of prenatal PCB exposure,
the heavier the girls were at age fourteen and their puberty was
statistically earlier. Boys with the higher prenatal exposure to
DDE also were fatter, but the age they entered puberty was
not affected. Scientists are now wondering if the epidemic of
childhood obesity may be partially caused by prenatal exposure
to endocrine disruptors?[3]

According to Sandra Steingraber, biologist and author of
Having Faith: An Ecologists Journey to Motherhood,

> "More profoundly, chemicals don't even have
> to cross the placenta to cause harm. Some lodge
> in the placenta and create injury there. For ex-
> ample, nicotine damages the placenta's amino
> acid transport system, which is used to ferry
> proteins from the mother's blood into the baby's.
> This helps explain why the babies of smoking
> mothers weight on an average of seven ounces
> less at birth. (Nicotine also passes through the
> placenta and into the body of the fetus.) Simi-
> larly, the industrial pollutants called PCBs alter
> the placenta's blood vessel in a way that reduces
> the flow, and nickel, a component of car exhaust,
> interferes with the placenta's ability to make and
> release hormones. In short, the placenta not only
> fails to keep the fetus out of harm's way, it cannot
> even prevent itself from being damaged. Like
> any other living tissue, it is fragile."[1]

It's hard to imagine we have arrived at a time in the history of our planet when every pregnant woman in the world
has hormone disrupting chemicals in her body, with total
disregard to race, gender or economic status. These chemicals
can either be transferred to the baby before birth or they can
enter during the time a mother is breast-feeding. A woman's
lifetime accumulation of toxics can even be passed on to her
fetus during pregnancy.

Chemicals and Birth Defects

When amniotic fluid from routine amniocentesis procedures was measured, it was found that 30 percent of women had detectable levels of the toxic chemicals PCBs, DDT and lindane. They also found detectable levels of estrogenic compounds such as phytoestrogens from food. The degree of concentration of in utero exposure is sufficient cause for great concern.

One chemical called DBP (dibutyl phthalate) is reported to cause severe birth defects in animals and sexual problems in human males. This chemical is widely used in shampoos, cosmetics, sunscreens, hair preparations, anti-perspirants and especially nail polish.[2]

Just think of all the women who either get their weekly manicures or paint their own fingernails. Just going to the beauty salon can be a toxic experience. Most beauty salons have little or no protection in the form of ventilation or air purification systems. Both customers and cosmetologists are at risk. One study concluded that cosmetologists had twice the risk of direct acting mutagens compared to dental workers. Mutagens can change the genetic code of a cell, and if sperm or eggs are affected, this can lead to birth defects. Genetic abnormalities can also result in spontaneous abortions. Cosmetologists who work full-time showed a higher rate of spontaneous abortion than women in other jobs. Again, this fact highlights the dangerous consequences of exposure to a range of toxic chemicals in daily use.

And what about pesticides? One example is Monsanto's best selling herbicide, Roundup that is a hormone-disruptor and is associated with birth defects in humans. Farm families that applied pesticides to their crops in Minnesota were studied to see if their elevated exposure to pesticides caused birth defects in their children. The study found that two kinds of pesticides — fungicides and the herbicide Roundup — were linked to statistically significant increases in birth defects. Roundup was linked to a 3-fold increase in neuro-developmental, showing up as attention deficit disorders.[3] Even one of our simplest pleasures, taking our daily shower, may pose serious health risks. A report by the Environmental Working Group and the US Public Interest Research Group warned pregnant women to avoid tap water and take shorter showers or baths to minimize exposure to chlorination by-products (CBPs), which places them at increased risk for miscarriages or birth defects. CBPs can be readily inhaled or absorbed through the skin. Using water filters for both drinking water and taking showers or non-chlorinated bottled water has now become a necessity.

Steroid hormones play a vital role in the womb by directing the development of the reproductive organs and as influencing the development of the thyroid gland, liver, immune system and brain. Critical times for breast development also occur before birth. This development requires an impeccable time sequence of events. Any alteration of the sequence can have disastrous and permanent consequences.

For example, on day 56 of human gestation, one particular hormone is required for the organs of the fetus to begin developing testicles. If the hormonal signal does not arrive, the fetus will lose the window of opportunity to develop into a male. If the timed sequence of hormone signals is disrupted for any reason, the development of the male reproductive organs can be skewed, resulting in undescended testicles or a number of other problems.

Females are also at risk. Chronic exposure to hormone disruptors during the embryo stage can result in functional loss of ovarian follicles in females. As women age, this can lead to decreased progesterone production, which results in estrogen dominance, PMS, endometriosis and miscarriages. Estrogen dominance can also contribute to a greater risk of breast cancer. Many other types of ovarian dysfunction can also be linked to these earlier exposures.

The effects of chemical and hormonal alterations are imprinted in the developing fetus like a ticking time bomb. Although it appears a healthy baby has been born, it takes many years, if not decades, for the real damage to become apparent.

What Studies Have Shown

Women who were infertile were 27 times more likely to have mixed or applied herbicides in the two years prior to attempting conception than women who were fertile.[1]

Children exposed to herbicides before one year of age were 10 times more likely to develop early persistent asthma.[2]

Phthalates are linked to preterm birth which helps to explain why the incidence of premature birth in the US has increased 23 percent since the early 1980's.[3]

PBDE levels high in breast milk of Texas women. The first study of polybrominated diphenyl ether (PBDE) contamination burdens in US breast milk finds levels 10 - 100 times higher than typical for Europe. Recent rapid increases in American PBDE levels are raising public health concerns because of the ability of this family of contaminants to interfere with thyroid control of brain development.[4]

Cadmium provokes estrogenic responses at extremely low levels of exposure. The effects include alterations in the uterus and mammary gland, increases in estrogen-controlled gene expression and, following exposure in the womb, increases in adult weight and the speed of reaching sexual maturity.[5]

Scientist from the US EPA finds that birth defects of several types are more common in babies born in wheat growing counties in the Great Plains. There is a theory about chlorophenoxy herbicides, like 2,4-D, causing birth defects in people.[6]

Nitrate is an endocrine disruptor. Because of the ubiquity of nitrate in manure and fertilizer runoff, this could have huge implications for water quality standards.[7]

Bisphenol-A is an environmental contaminant causing a genetic error in human DNA which leads to spontaneous miscarriages and birth defects, including Down Syndrome. BPA also has been found at low levels in water supplies.[8]

Mother's milk is considered the perfect food. And, indeed, it is an elixir that bestows untold benefits to the newborn. A lactating mother transfers to her child a temporary immunity to the various diseases she overcame during her lifetime. It is also crucial to establishing the infant's permanent immune system. Breast fed babies have fewer allergies and breast milk acts to speed up intestinal growth. Elements in breast milk also turn on certain genes in the cells of the small intestine which send protein signals to developing immune tissues. Special sugars in human milk feed the growing intestinal flora. These sugars, which are not found in commercial infant formulas, provide food for the beneficial bacteria in the colon. No infant formula that can even come close to the miracle of mother's milk but, even breast milk is not immune from a toxic environment. Low doses of environmental toxins are fat-soluble and are stored in fatty tissue, including breast tissue. The chemicals stored in mother's fat are not released in significant amounts except during breast-feeding. So, while breast feeding lessens the mother's body burden of toxic chemicals, a human baby breast-fed for six months receives five times the allowable daily limit of PCBs set by international health standards for a 150-pound adult. A woman passes half of her lifetime accumulation of dioxins and PCBs on to her child when she nurses for just six months. The most consistent dietary predictor of PCB concentration in breast tissue is fish consumption.

One class of chemicals called polybrominated flame retardants (PBDEs) used in many different types of plastics and plastic-containing products, are known thyroid disruptors that are both persistent and bioaccumulative. When they leach out of the plastics they quickly find their way into the biosphere. Since the 1970s, PBDEs have increased more than 50-fold in breast milk.

Mothers Milks Turns Sour

If breast milk were regulated like infant formula, it would commonly violate FDA levels for poisonous substances in food.[1] In spite of the contamination of breast milk, it is still considered by both scientists and pediatricians to be the most ideal food for infants. The present theory is higher rates of chemical exposure from breast milk are less significant than the smaller amounts that coming from in utero exposure. Even though more chemicals may be transferred to the nursing infant, exposure while in the womb is considered more potentially disrupting. When it comes to breast feeding, there is unanimous agreement the benefits far outweigh the risks. Don't ever give up on Mother Nature.

To sum it up, the womb experience is now fraught with many invisible dangers. The undeniable toxic exposure in utero to synthetic hormones, petrochemicals, organochlorines found in pesticides, fungicides, herbicides and insecticides, along with the new members to the club such as phthalates, nonylphenol and bisphenol-A, pose a grave risk to the developing fetus. The effects to the fetus' developing brain, immune system, reproductive system, endocrine system and behavioral development may not be observed until puberty or beyond. These man made chemicals tweak the genes into mutations that can lead to numerable possible health problems, some of them life-threatening. Certainly the quality of a person's life can be seriously jeopardized.

The other tricky bit is it's not only the kind of hormone disrupting chemicals introduced into a fetus' world, but also the timing of exposure. If certain chemicals arrive on the scene at critical moments of a fetus' growth, then that particular function can be permanently compromised and impaired for life.

Without testing for these toxins, a mother has no idea what might be poisoning her baby.

When it comes to breast cancer and other reproductive cancers, we now know the seeds planted during that tender womb time, as well as the breast-feeding period, can be setting a course in motion predisposing girls to breast cancer as adults (and for boys, it's prostate and testicular cancer). We must be aware of these dangers so we can take all the possible precautions to protect our unborn children and infants.

Chapter 5
Soy Infant Formulas
A Wolf in Sheep's Clothing!

The humble soybean has had a meteoric rise to fame and fortune in Western countries during the last decade. Like any high profile rock star or movie idol, lots of media hype and multi-million dollar marketing efforts have been essential to make this bean a household name. Making the soybean into a legitimate infant formula product has been a well-planned and expensive process. It certainly appears to have paid off since it is estimated that soy-based formulas accounts for $750 million of the $3 billion baby formulas market. Soy is still a star on the way up since sales have more than doubled in the last ten years.

According to Naomi Baumslag, clinical professor of pediatrics at Georgetown University Medical College, "Only 50 percent of newborns today suckle at the mother's breast even once. After six months, the number has fallen to only one mother in five. Often mothers for the sake of convenience plunk soy bottles into the infant's mouth."[1] In fact, nearly 20 percent of infants worldwide are fed soy formula, with 750,000 US infants receiving soy formula every year.

There certainly seems a lot more going on behind the scenes when it comes to the truth about soy formulas. What has finally been revealed is quite shocking.

Something very troubling began to be noticed in Puerto Rico twenty years ago. In 1982 pediatric endocrinologists reported an increase in the incidence of breast development in girls as young as two years old. In one study approximately 68 percent of the cases (85 out of 130) studied experienced the onset of sexual development before they were 18 months old.

Soy and Hormones

Many causes were investigated and eventually one of the culprits was found. Soy-based infant formulas! It was discovered the phytoestrogens in soy formulas were stimulating this early development.

A 1997 *Lancet* study showed soy has glycosides of genistein and daidzein or plant based chemicals mimicking estrogen. They possess a wide range of hormonal and non-hormonal activities. The daily exposure of infants who consume soy formulas was 6-11 times higher than adults consuming soy foods. The blood concentration of these hormones was 13,000 to 22,000 times higher than estrogen in the blood. The authors of the article speculate this concentration may be sufficient to exert biological effects, whereas the contribution from breast-milk or cow-milk is negligible.[2]

There is now mounting evidence the increase in early on-set of puberty occurring in North America, Australia, the UK, and Europe, as well many other countries, coincides with the record level sales of soy formula. Many questions have now been raised. Just what are the long-term risks associated with premature sexuallity?

There is still debate over whether or not premature development progresses to precocious puberty, but there is evidence from several studies showing it does increase the chance of early puberty. A higher incidence of ovarian cysts has also been found in girls developing breasts at an early age. The earlier the onset of menarche, the greater the lifetime risk of breast cancer. The early incidence of ovarian cysts is an established risk factor in the later development of ovarian cancer. Could these excessively high levels of estrogenic hormones predispose girls to serious hormonal imbalances including breast cancer later in life?

Soy's estrogenic exposure may also be putting little boys at risk. Infant boys go through a "testosterone tide" during the first six months of their lives, when they normally have testosterone levels nearly equal to those of mature men. This early surge of male hormones programs the reproductive system, brain and other organs to take on male characteristics at puberty. Researchers are now wondering whether the feeding of estrogen-rich soy formula to infant boys interferes with this process. They believe soy formula is the explanation for a syndrome, becoming more and more frequent, wherein the male sexual organs do not properly develop at puberty.

The *New Zealand Medical Journal* found soy-based infant formula may adversely affect hormonal development in neonatal infants and should not be sold commercially. Since soy is the richest source of phytoestrogens, a plant form of the female hormone estrogen, neonatal infants are particularly vulnerable. The *New Zealand Medical Journal* cautioned there is insufficient research on the long-term health effects of phytoestrogens, therefore warranting a ban on the nonprescription sale of soy formula.[3]

According to Dr. Mike Fitzpatrick, a New Zealand toxicologist, babies fed exclusively on soy formula receive the estrogenic equivalent of at least five birth control pills per day. As a result of this evidence, both the British and New Zealand governments have issued warnings on the use of soy infant formula.

If soy's estrogenic effect wasn't bad enough, there are other serious problems with soy formulas. Both soy and soy formulas initiate thyroid disease in infants. Feeding infants soy formulas exposes them to high levels of isoflavones, which are potent anti-thyroid agents. This poses significant risks to normal growth and development.

Soy Warnings

Lynn Goldman, MD, MPH, Professor of Environmental Health Science, *Johns Hopkins University Bloomberg School of Public Health*, also voiced concerns. A report published in *Cancer Research* found that genistein, one of the isoflavones in soy, was more carcinogenic (dose adjusted for estrogen potency) than the synthetic estrogen DES when exposure occurred during "critical periods of differentiation," such as during infancy. Medical professionals insisted DES was safe for pregnant women until they discovered many years later the women whose mothers took DES suffered from very high rates of cervical cancer. The authors of the *Cancer Research* study concluded ". . . the use of soy-based infant formulas in the absence of medical necessity and the marketing of soy products designed to appeal to children should be closely examined."

A policy statement of the *Royal College of Australian Physicians* includes their comments about soy formulas.[4] The rationale for the use of soy formula has been the assumption that soy protein is less allergic than cow's milk. This is not the case. Soy protein can cause intolerance reactions with gastrointestinal symptoms and acute allergic reactions. In fact, up to 40 percent of infants intolerant of cow's milk also develop soy protein intolerance. Soy can cause a loss of vitamins, minerals and trace elements from the gut. High aluminum content has also been documented in soy formula. It has over 1000 percent more aluminum than conventional milk based formulas. Infants fed soy formula also had lower levels of antibodies in response to routine immunizations and more infections than those fed human milk or cow's milk formula, leading to compromise immunity.

The soybean plant lifts up manganese in the soil and concentrates it. Its use in soy-based infant formula can result in as many as 200 times the level found in natural breast milk, thus, overloading an infants body. New research suggests high concentrations of manganese found in soybean-based baby formula can lead to brain damage in infants and altered behaviors in adolescents. Newborn infants exposed to high levels of manganese may be predisposed to neurological problems.[5]

The experts are asking very important question these days about soy. Why deprive the newborn infants of perfectly good breast milk - a nutritionally superior food in every way for the baby and feed them soy beans which have serious adverse hormonal effects. Without a doubt, soy formula is one of the worst foods possibly fed to both infants and children.

So, now that the beans have been spilled about soy formulas, milk might appear as a better alternative. Unfortunately that is not the case. Since commercial, pasteurized milk is loaded with antibiotics, bovine growth hormones and a whole host of allergic and indigestible ingredients, it poses many health problems for the developing infant as well.

However, while there is no way to create a formula equal to breast milk, there are steps that can be taken to improve upon the standard formulas are available and provide the key nutritional support for a rapidly growing infant. The best solution is to learn to make truly safe, beneficial and nutritious infant formulas.

Home-made Baby Formulas

The following formulas take into account the specific nutritional needs of an infant. Sally Fallon, director of the Weston A. Price Foundation and author of *Nourishing Traditions* has compiled balanced, healthy and nutritious recipes for those infants requiring an infant formula.

Milk-based Formula (Makes 36 ounces)

This milk-based formula takes into account human milk is richer in whey, lactose, vitamin C, niacin, and long-chain polyunsaturated fatty acids compared to cow's milk but leaner in casein (milk protein). The addition of gelatin to cow's milk formula will make it more digestible for the infant. Use only truly expeller-expressed oils in the formula recipes, otherwise they may lack vitamin E.

The ideal milk for baby, if it cannot be breast fed, is organic, whole raw milk from old-fashioned cows, certified free of disease and fed on green pasture. If the only choice available to you is commercial milk, choose whole milk, preferably organic and unhomogenized and culture it with a kefier culture to restore enzymes.

> 2 c whole milk, preferably unprocessed, unpastuerized milk from pasture-fed cows
> 1/4 c homemade liquid whey (See recipe for whey, below)
> 4 tbsp lactose (2 or more tablespoons good quality cream (not ultra-pasteurized), more if you are using milk from Holstein cows
> 1 tsp cod liver oil
> 1 tsp expeller-expressed sunflower oil
> 1 tsp extra virgin olive oil
> 2 tsp coconut oil
> 2 tsp Frontier brand nutritional yeast flakes
> 2 tsp gelatin
> 1 7/8 c filtered water
> 1 tsp. acerola powder

Add gelatin to water and heat gently until gelatin is dissolved. Place all ingredients in a very clean glass or stainless steel container and mix well. To serve, pour 6 to 8 ounces into a very clean glass bottle, attach nipple and set in a pan of simmering water. Heat until warm but not hot to the touch, shake bottle well and feed baby. (Never heat formula in a microwave oven!) If you are using the Lact-Aid, mix all ingredients well in a blender.

Variation: Goat Milk Formula

Although goat milk is rich in fat, it must be used with caution in infant feeding as it lacks folic acid and is low in vitamin B12, both of which are essential to the growth and development of the infant. Inclusion of nutritional yeast to provide folic acid is essential. To compensate for low levels of vitamin B12, add 2 teaspoons frozen organic raw chicken liver, finely grated to the batch of formula. Be sure to begin egg-yolk feeding at four months.

Liver-based Formulas (Makes about 36 ounces)

This liver-based formula also mimics the nutrient profile of mother's milk. It is extremely important to include coconut oil in this formula, as it is the only ingredient that provides the special medium-chain saturated fats found in mother's milk. As with the milk-based formula, all oils should be truly expeller-expressed.

3 3/4 cups homemade beef or chicken broth
2 oz organic liver, cut into small pieces
1 tsp bifidobacterium infantis
1/4 c homemade liquid whey (See recipe for whey, p. 83)
1 tbsp coconut oil
1 tsp cod liver oil
1 tsp unrefined sunflower oil
2 tsp extra virgin olive oil
1 tsp acerola powder

Simmer liver gently in broth until the meat is cooked through. Liquefy using a handheld blender or in a food processor. When the liver broth has cooled, stir in remaining ingredients. Store in a very clean glass or stainless steel container. To serve, stir formula well and pour 6 to 8 ounces in a very clean glass bottle. Attach a clean nipple and set in a pan of simmering water until formula is warm but not hot to the touch, shake well and feed to baby.

Fortified Commercial Formula (Makes about 35 ounces)

This stop gap formula can be used in emergencies, or when the ingredients for homemade formula are unavailable. 1 cup Mead Johnson low-iron, milk-based powdered formula:

29 oz filtered water (3 5/8 cups)
1 large egg yolk from an organic egg, cooked 3 1/2 minutes
(See recipe for egg yolk, below)
1 tsp cod liver oil

Place all ingredients in a blender or food processor and blend thoroughly. Place 6-8 ounces in a very clean glass bottle. Attach a clean nipple to the bottle and set in a pan of simmering water until formula is warm but not hot to the touch, shake well and feed to baby.

Egg Yolk for Baby

Egg yolk should be baby's first solid food, starting at 4 months, whether baby is breast fed or formula-fed. Egg yolks from pastured hens will contain the special long-chain fatty acids so critical for the optimal development of the brain and nervous system. The whites may cause an allergic reaction and should not be given to baby until he is at least one year old.

1 organic egg from a pasture-fed hen
1/2 tsp grated raw organic liver, frozen for 14 days (optional)
Boil egg for 3 1/2 minutes. Place in a bowl and peel off shell. Remove egg white and discard. Yolk should be soft and warm, not hot, with its enzyme content intact.

If you wish to add liver, grate on the small holes of a grater while frozen. Allow to warm up and stir into egg yolk.

Homemade Whey (Makes about 5 cups)

Homemade whey is easy to make from good quality plain yogurt, or from raw or cultured milk. You will need a large strainer that rests over a bowl.

If you are using yogurt, place 2 quarts in the strainer lined with a tea towel. Cover with a plate and leave at room temperature overnight. The whey will drip out into the bowl. Place whey in clean glass jars and store in the refrigerator.

If you are using raw or cultured milk, place 2 quarts of the milk in a glass container and leave at room temperature for 2-4 days until the milk separates into curds and whey. Pour into the strainer lined with a tea towel and cover with a plate. Leave at room temperature overnight. The whey will drip out into the bowl. Store in clean glass jars in the refrigerator.

Premature Infants

If your baby is premature, one additional area of fortification is free amino acids, most notably taurine. This nutrient is also critical for infant development and is found in human milk but not in cow's milk. Although many formulas add some taurine, it has been shown formula-fed infants have lower levels of taurine in their blood than breast fed infants do, even when the formula has added taurine.

For further information contact:

The Weston A. Price Foundation
Phone: 202.333.HEAL
Email: WestonAPrice@msn.com
http://www.westonaprice.org
To find any ingredient listed in any of the formulas contact:
Radiant Life - 888-593-8333
http://www.4radiantlife.com

Our home is our refuge from the outer world. It's the one reliable place where we can retreat into safety and comfort. We like to think we can close the front door and all will be well. In some cases it may be true, but when it comes to the world of toxic concoctions, our homes are really havens for a wide variety dangerous chemicals and hormone disruptors. Harboring such intruders can put our children in harm's way.

Daily we swish, wipe, rub, wash, and spray our way through dozens of cleaning products in an attempt to maintain a spotless, dust-free, pestless home. We're assured by smiling, dancing TV homemakers we're doing the right thing.

Our cupboards are tightly packed, our laundry is fully stocked and the cabinet beneath our kitchen and bathroom sink is ready for any mishap.

Our private world is pristine! Well, not exactly.

Here's a troubling statistic. It is an accepted fact the indoor air can be up to 10 times more polluted than the outside air.

Our energy efficient homes keep out the cold and the heat in. What also stays inside are all the chemicals is the constant outgassing from the building materials, carpets, plastics etc.

Have you ever really looked at the ingredients in all these products? It's a tongue-twisting experience to even attempt to pronounce them. We have been so successfully indoctrinated into the world of chemicals, people rarely, stop to give some serious thought as to what these chemicals are and what they might be doing to our health.

Many of these chemicals are carcinogens and endocrine disruptors. During the first five years of life, children are exposed to the same levels of endocrine disruptors that used to be considered safe lifetime exposures for seventy-year-old adults.

Children are more vulnerable to the various chemicals floating around homes and other buildings because they are exposed to more toxic substances than adults. Children inhale twenty-three times more air, drink three times as much water, and eat two to three times as much food per pound of body weight as do adults. They also have three times more surface area per pound than adults. These differences mean children have greater rates of exposure to environmental chemicals than adults.

Also, infants and toddlers put more contaminants in their mouths. The way they handle food could contribute to 20-80 percent of their total dietary intake of pesticides. They also absorb chemicals through their skin, gastrointestinal tract, and lungs better than adults. They crawl around on the floor where dust, especially in carpeting, has been shown by scientific data to be a serious route of exposure to chemical residues, many of which are tracked into the house from our shoes.

Young infants have poorly developed systems for detoxifying chemicals, so the chemicals they are exposed to tend to stay in their bodies. Certain man-made chemicals may be particularly damaging right after birth. They may interfere with the hormones and other substances that send out signals normally controlling development. Hormone disrupting chemicals can more easily influence the development of the rapidly developing central nervous, immune, respiratory and reproductive systems.

Indoor Health Concerns

Solvents like benzene, xylene, toluene and styrene (Styrofoam), can lower testosterone and sperm levels, contribute to abortions, birth defects, asthma, nose congestion and adversely affect the blood and heart.[1]

Studies indicate chemicals in moth balls and deodorants (dichlrobenzene) were found in the urine of 96 percent of children in Arkansas.[2]

Leukemia is several times more likely in children if pesticides are used in and around a home.[3]

A non-occupational chemical exposure study showed households contained 5 to 20 different pesticides. This does not include the other chemicals in the air.[4]

The level of pesticides in the air is nearly four times greater at 5 to 10 inches above the floor, than it is at 24 inches. This puts toddlers at risk.[5]

Chemicals released from hot Teflon pots, microwaved foods, disinfectants, deodorizers, oven cleaners, carpet cleaners, foods and cooking odors, hair or ironing sprays etc. all can contribute to indoor air and body pollution.[6]

The Consumer Product Safety Commission reported 150 common household chemicals have been linked to allergies, birth defects, cancer and psychological abnormalities.[7]

The Danger Is Within - David's Story

When he was two weeks old, David passed out while breast-feeding. Rushed to the emergency room by his panicked mother, he recovered consciousness, but the doctors couldn't figure out the cause. Within the next six to eight months, David passed out numerous times and was in and out of the hospital where he was often hooked up to a respirator. His parents were counseled to prepare for David's death. Doctors pronounced his case hopeless, and said spending more money on hospital care (they had already spent close to 300,000 dollars) was useless.

No doctor could pinpoint the cause of David's fainting episodes, but his mother was on a mission to find it.

After the mainstream medical caregivers gave up on David, his mom hired a full-time pediatric nurse and turned to alternative medicine. A homeopath suggested keeping a diary of David's symptoms. This experience was revelatory. Every Tuesday David ended up in the hospital. How could that be?

The journal showed that on Tuesdays, his mom cleaned the house. Thinking that cleaning might contribute to David's problems, she didn't clean the house for two weeks and David slept through the night for the first time in his young life. David's doctor thought the connection to cleaning was a coincidence, so his mom cleaned the house again and David ended up in the emergency room.

Now on the path of some answers, his mom looked up every chemical listed on the bottles of her cleaning products, read every book she could find and contacted experts in healthy homes. She soon realized her son had all the symptoms of environmental illness from exposure to toxic chemicals in commercial cleaning products she used.

His mom began to remove all the poisons from her home to cure her son in the process. She was stunned to discover there were very few pure and healthy products to substitute for the toxic chemical she'd used to "clean" her home. Determined to find substitutes for toxic chemicals, she made her own cleansers. Her investigation and research led to the family creating a successful company now manufacturing a line of natural household cleaners for those who suffer from allergies, asthma and chemical sensitivities.

David is now eight years old and thriving because his family was fortunate to discover the chemicals that make him so deathly sick.

So, you think you couldn't possibly survive without all those house-cleaning products? It should be obvious by now one of the best ways to improve the quality of your indoor air is by cleaning without toxic chemicals. There are many companies who specialize in safe, non-toxic cleaning products. Most of them are found in health food stores or progressive supermarkets.

Another alternative is to return to the days of your grandmother and make your own. If you're feeling adventurous, you may want to try some of the following recipes. They are effective, simple and very cheap. As an added bonus, ounce for ounce homemade cleaning formulas cost about one-tenth the price of their commercial counterparts.

The Basic Ingredients

Baking Soda

A commonly available mineral full of many cleaning attributes, baking soda is made from soda ash, and is slightly alkaline (it's pH is around 8.1; 7 is neutral). It neutralizes acid-based odors in water and absorbs odors from the air. Sprinkled on a damp sponge or cloth, baking soda can be used as a gentle non abrasive cleanser for kitchen counter tops, sinks, bathtubs, ovens, and fiberglass. You can eliminate perspiration odors and neutralize the smell of many chemicals by adding a cup per load to the laundry. It is a useful air freshener and carpet deodorizer.

Washing Soda

A chemical neighbor of baking soda, washing soda (sodium carbonate) is much more strongly alkaline, with a pH of 11. It releases no harmful fumes and is far safer than a commercial solvent formula. Wear gloves when using it because it is caustic.

Washing soda cuts grease, cleans petroleum oil, removes wax or lipstick and neutralizes odors in the same way baking soda does. Don't use it on fiberglass, aluminum or waxed floors—unless you intend to remove the wax.

White Vinegar and Lemon Juice

White vinegar and lemon juice are acidic. They neutralize alkaline substances such as scale from hard water. Acids dissolve gummy buildup, eat away tarnish, and remove dirt from wood surfaces.

Liquid Soaps and Detergent

Liquid soaps and detergents are necessary for cutting grease, but they are not the same. Soap is made from fats and lye. Detergents are synthetic materials. Unlike soap, detergents are designed specifically so they don't react with hard water minerals and cause soap scum. If you have hard water, buy a biodegradable detergent without perfumes. If you have soft water you can use liquid soap.

Disinfectants

There are many essential oils, such as lavender, clove, and tea tree oil (an excellent natural fungicide) are very antiseptic, as is grapefruit seed extract. Use one teaspoon of essential oil to 2 cups of water in a spray bottle (make sure to avoid eyes). A grapefruit seed extract spray can be made by adding 20 drops of extract to a quart of water.

The Alchemist in the Kitchen

The following are some cleaning product formulas. They

are so simple to make using the basic ingredients. With very little time, you can concoct some of the best cleaning products ever! They can replace all the toxic versions. It's also a great project to teach to the kids!

Creamy Soft Scrubber

Simply pour about 1/2 cup of baking soda into a bowl and add enough liquid detergent to make a texture like frosting. Scoop the mixture onto a sponge and wash the surface. This is the perfect recipe for cleaning the bathtub because it rinses easily and doesn't leave grit.

Add 1 teaspoon of vegetable glycerin to the mixture and store in a sealed glass jar, to keep the product moist. Otherwise just make as much as you need for the task.

Window Cleaner

1/4 - 1/2-teaspoon liquid detergent
3 tablespoons vinegar
2 cups water
Spray bottle

Put all the ingredients into a spray bottle, shake it up a bit and use as you would a commercial brand. The soap in this recipe is important. It cuts the wax residue from the commercial brands you might have used in the past.

Oven Cleaner

1 cup or more baking soda
Water
A squirt or two of liquid detergent

Sprinkle water generously over the bottom of the oven, then cover the grime with enough baking soda to make the surface totally white. Sprinkle some more water over the top. Let the mixture set overnight. You can easily wipe up the grease the next morning because the grime will have loosened. When you have cleaned up the worst of the mess, dab a bit of liquid detergent or soap on a sponge, and wash the remaining residue from the oven. If this recipe doesn't work for you it is probably because you didn't use enough baking soda and/or water.

All-purpose Spray Cleaner

1/2 tsp. washing soda
A dab of liquid soap
2 cups hot tap water

Combine the ingredients in a spray bottle and shake until the washing soda has dissolved. Apply and wipe off with a sponge or rag.

Furniture Polish

1/2 teaspoon oil, such as olive (or jojoba, a liquid wax)
1/4 cup vinegar or fresh lemon juice

Mix the ingredients in a glass jar. Dab a soft rag into the solution and wipe onto wood surfaces. Cover the glass jar and store indefinitely.

Vinegar Deodorizer

Keep a clean spray bottle filled with 5 percent vinegar in your kitchen and bathroom for cleaning. The smell of vinegar dissipates within a few hours. Undiluted vinegar is also great for cleaning the toilet rim. Just spray it on and wipe off.

Mold Killers

Nothing natural works for mold and mildew as well as this spray. It's effective on everything from a moldy ceiling a musty bureau, a musty rug, or moldy shower curtain. Tea tree oil is expensive and a little goes a very long way. The smell of tea tree oil is very strong, but it will dissipate in a few days. This formula will make about 2 cups and has an indefinite shelf life.

2 teaspoons tea tree oil
2 cups water

Combine in a spray bottle, shake to blend, and spray on problem areas. Do not rinse.

Vinegar Spray

Undiluted vinegar reportedly kills 82 percent of mold. Pour some white distilled vinegar straight into a spray bottle, spray on the moldy area, and let set without rinsing.

In our society looking good, smelling sweet and feeling soft and smooth keeps us spending billions of dollars annually. The very commercial products we spray, splash, wash with, rub on, and get pretty with harbor a more sinister side. Men in white lab coats whip up chemical concoctions are designed to be used on our body. While we naively accept advertising enticements, most people are unaware that personal care products are part of an unregulated industry, which incorporates known carcinogenic and hormone disrupting chemicals.

Most women use a wide range of cosmetics on a regular basis. It has been estimated an average woman may have up to 400 exposures to chemicals each week from the products she uses. Many of these chemicals find their way into the bodies of children. Many more chemicals are found in commercial baby and children's personal care products.

The skin is not a barrier but rather a gatekeeper. Whatever is applied to the skin is usually absorbed and journeys into the blood stream. When commercial personal care products are rubbed into bodies of infants and children, a long list of foreign and sometimes toxic chemicals also enter the body.

Newborn skin is more permeable to topically applied agents than adult skin, making systemic toxicity much greater in newborns.

In the United States, cosmetics are second only to household cleaners as the leading poisons of children.

Journalist Joel Bleifus of the *Chicago Tribune* wrote the following expose' providing an inside peek in the hidden world of personal care products.

> Do you use toothpaste, shampoo, sunscreen, body lotion, body talc, makeup, or hair dye? These are among the personal care products the American consumer has been led to believe are safe but are

often contaminated with carcinogenic by products, or contain substances regularly reacting to form potent carcinogens during storage and use.

Consumers regularly assume these products are not harmful because they believe they are approved for safety by the Food and Drug Administration (FDA). Although the FDA classifies cosmetics (dividing them into 13 categories); it does not regulate them. An FDA document posted on the agency's World Wide Web home page explains, "A cosmetic manufacturer may use any ingredient or raw material and market the final product without government approval." (This is with the exception of seven known toxins, such as hexachlorophene, mercury compounds, and chloroform). Should the FDA deem a product a danger to public health, it has the power to pull a cosmetic product from the shelves. In many of these cases, the FDA has failed to do so, while evidence mounts some of the most common cosmetic ingredients may double as deadly carcinogens.

Example of products with potential carcinogens are: Clairol "Nice and Easy" hair color, which releases carcinogenic formaldehyde as well as Cocamide DEA (a substance which can be contaminated with carcinogenic nitrosamines or react to produce a nitrosamine during storage or use); Vidal Sassoon shampoo (which like the hair dye, contains Cocamide DEA); Cover Girl makeup contains TEA (which is also associated with carcinogenic nitrosamines); Crest toothpaste which contains titanium dioxide, saccharin, and FD&C Blue #1 (known carcinogens).

One of the cosmetic toxins consumer advocates are most concerned about is nitrosamine, which contaminates a wide variety of cosmetic products. In the 1970s nitrosamine contamination of cooked bacon and other nitrite-treated meats became a public-health issue. The food industry, which is more strictly regulated than the cosmetic industry, has since drastically lowered the amount of nitrosamines found in processed meats. Today nitrosamines contaminate cosmetics at significantly higher levels than were once contained in bacon.

The FDA has long known nitrosamines in cosmetics pose a risk to public health. On April 10, 1979, FDA commissioner Donald Kennedy called on the cosmetic industry to "take immediate measures to eliminate, to the extent possible, NDELA [a potent nitrosamine] and any other N-nitrosamine from cosmetic products." Since the warning, however, cosmetic manufacturers have done little to remove N-nitrosamines from their products and the FDA has done even less to monitor them.[1]

What about Sunscreens?

Six frequently used UVA and UVB sunscreens were tested by the Institute of Pharmacology and Toxicology at the University of Zurich, Switzerland, for their estrogenic effect.[2]

The chemicals analyzed were: benzophenone-3 (Bp-3), homosalate (HMS), 4-methyl-benzylidene camphor (4-MBC), octyl-methoxycinnamate (OMC), octyl-dimethyl-PABA (OD-PABA), and butyl-methoxydibenzoylmethane (B-MDM).

What do the first five ingredients all have in common?

They were all estrogen mimicking chemicals. The researchers concluded there was enough evidence of estrogenicity for further studies to be warranted.

Are you sure you want to slather estrogenic sunscreens on your children? Instead, look for safe non-toxic sunscreen products.

From day one, a newborn is introduced to a huge array of chemicals being applied to its little body in the name of tender loving care. Are you aware you might be putting your children's mental, emotional and physical health at risk each time you wash their hair, splash around in bubble bath, brush their teeth, powder their bottoms, apply moisturizers or use baby wipes? Are these products safe and non-toxic?

The word *nontoxic* appears on many consumer products but it is misleading. According to the federal regulatory definition, *nontoxic doesn't* mean "not at all toxic" or "absolutely safe". It means that up to half of the laboratory animals exposed to the product through ingestion of inhalation died within two weeks. A product can also be called *nontoxic* if no serious (immediate) damage occurred through eye or skin contact. These tests reflect only short-term health effects that may be associated with the product. Long-term or chronic effects are not considered."[34]

The following are some of the most daily used hazardous ingredients found in personal care products marketed to both children and adults.

> **Alcohol, Isopopyl (SD-40):** a very drying and irritating solvent and dehydrator that strips the skin's moisture and natural immune barrier, making you more vulnerable to bacteria, molds and viruses. It is made from propylene, a petroleum derivative found in many skin and hair products, fragrance, antibacterial hand washes, shellac and antifreeze. It can act as a "carrier" accelerating the penetration of harmful chemicals into the skin. It may cause headaches, dizziness, mental depression, nausea, vomiting and coma. Fatal ingested dose is one ounce.

DEA (diethanolamine), MEA (monoethanolamine), TEA (triethanolamine): hormone disrupting chemicals can form cancer-causing nitrates and nitrosamines. Although restricted in Europe due to its carcinogenic effects, Americans may be exposed 10-20 times per day. Used to create "foam" in products like shampoo, shaving cream and bubble bath.

DMD Hydantoin and Urea (Imidazolidinyl): Two of many preservatives that often release formaldehyde which can cause joint pain, skin reactions, allergies, depression, headaches, chest pains, ear infections, chronic fatigue, dizziness and loss of sleep. Exposure may also irritate the respiratory system, trigger heart palpitations or asthma, and aggravate colds and coughs. Other possible side effects include weakening the immune system and cancer.

FD&C Color Pigments: Synthetic colors made from coal tar containing heavy metal salts that deposit toxins onto the skin, causing skin sensitivity and irritation. Absorption of certain colors can cause depletion of oxygen in the body and death. Animal studies have shown almost all of them to be carcinogenic.

Fragrances: Fragrance on a label can indicate the presence of up to four thousand separate ingredients, many toxic or carcinogenic. Symptoms reported to the FDA include headaches, dizziness, allergic rashes, skin discoloration, violent coughing, vomiting, and skin irritation.

Clinical observation proves fragrances can affect the central nervous system, causing depression, hyperactivity, irritability, inability to cope and other behavioral changes.

Mineral Oil: Petroleum by-product that coats the skin like plastic, clogging the pores. Interferes with the skin's ability to eliminate toxins, promotes acne and other disorders. Slows down skin function and cell development, resulting in premature aging. Baby oil is 100 per cent mineral oil.

Polyethylene glycol (PEG): Potentially carcinogenic petroleum ingredient can alter and reduce the skin's natural moisture factor. This could increase the appearance of aging and leave you more vulnerable to bacteria. Used in cleansers to dissolve oil and grease, and used in caustic spray-on oven cleaners.

Propylene Glycol(PG) and Butylene Glycol: Petroleum plastics which act as 'surfactant' (wetting agents and solvents). They easily penetrate the skin and can weaken protein and cellular structure. PG is strong enough to remove barnacles from boats! The EPA considers PG so toxic it requires workers to wear protective gloves, clothing and goggles and to dispose of any PG solutions by burying them in the ground. Since PG penetrates the skin so quickly, the EPA warns against skin contact to prevent consequences such as brain, liver and kidney abnormalities. There isn't even a warning label on products such as stick deodorants, where the concentration is greater than in most industrial applications.

Sodium Lauryl Sulfate (SLS) and Sodium Laureth Sulfate (SLES): Detergents and surfactants pose serious health threats. Used in car washes, garage floor, cleaners, engine degreasers and 90% of personal-care products. Animals exposed to SLS experienced eye damage, depression, labored breathing, diarrhea, severe skin irritation and even death. Young eyes may not develop properly if exposed to SLS because proteins are dissolved. SLS may also damage the skin's immune system by causing layers to separate and inflame. When combined with other chemicals, SLS can be transformed into nitrosamines. The body may retain SLS for up to five days during which it may enter and maintain residual levels in the heart, liver, lungs and brain.

Tricolsan: A synthetic "antibacterial" ingredient with a chemical structure similar to Agent Orange. The EPA registers it as a pesticide with great risk to both human health and the environment. It is classified as a class of chemicals suspected of causing cancer in humans. Its manufacturing process may produce dioxin, a powerful hormone disrupting chemical with toxic effects measured in parts per trillion. (equivalent to one drop in 300 Olympic-size swimming pools) Internally, it will damage the liver, kidneys and lungs and will cause paralysis, suppression of immune function, brain hemorrhages and heart problems. Tufts University School of Medicine says that triclosan is capable of forcing the emergence of 'super bugs' that it cannot kill. It is widely used in toothpastes and household products.

Almost every sponge now sold in U.S. supermarkets is impregnated with a synthetic disinfectant—usually triclosan.

There is no doubt commercial personal care products have no place in one's life. Certainly, they should never be use on or around children. You have a choice. There are many organic, chemical-free baby and children's products readily available. Remember, you can quite easily make your own natural products.

The many risks present in our world may seem overwhelming. The good news is when it comes to our own personal space in and around our home, there are many ways to create a cleaner environment offering greater protection. The following are some guidelines to help lessen the toxic load. If you are thinking of becoming pregnant or are presently pregnant or breast-feeding, these suggestions will support you and your baby's health and well-being. In fact, the whole family will benefit. Little changes can make a world of difference. You may prefer to take baby steps when making the transition from toxic to non-toxic. Whatever way you choose to incorporate reducing toxic exposure, make it the one you will commit to.

1. Eliminate all commercial household cleaning products and replace with natural, non-toxic cleaning products.

2. Avoid all pesticides, herbicides, insecticides, and fungicides. Keep them out of your home and off your lawns. Use organic alternatives.

3. Avoid all commercial personal care products including shampoos, conditioners, baby shampoos, soaps, bubble baths, toothpaste, moisturizers, air fresheners, deodorants, hairspray and nail polish. They all contain hormone disrupting ingredients. Find organic, chemical free products.

4. If you dry clean your clothes, be sure to air them outside for at least 24 hours.

5. Use glass, ceramic or stainless steel containers for foods and beverages.

6. Avoid plastic packaging and plastic cling wrap, especially in the microwave.

7. Dust tracked in on shoes has high levels of pesticides and lead. Whenever possible, take off your shoes before entering the house or wipe your feet on a good doormat. Vacuum carpets once or twice a week. Be sure to wipe all surfaces regularly.

8. Include a regular sauna, either dry or wet, as part of a detoxification program. The skin is a major organ of detoxification and toxins are released as we sweat. In recent years saunas have become recognized as one of the few methods to remove toxic chemicals from the body, particularly when they are stored in the fat cells. It has been shown chlorinated pesticides, herbicides and PCBs have been successfully eliminated from the body. With regular use of saunas, a good proportion of environmental toxins can be eliminated from the body. In this way, women can reduce their toxic burden and the toxic burden that may get passed on to their baby.

9. Seek out a competent holistic practitioner, such as an alternative medical doctor, naturopath, nutritionist, chiropractor, or an oriental medical practitioner to help assess your health and create a program to help to detoxify and heal your body.

10. Become an activist for change. What recently occurred in Quebec, Montreal is an inspiration for what other communities can do. In 2002, Quebec announced new pesticide laws stating

that no pesticides will be mixed with fertilizers or used in schools, daycare centers or on pubic lands including hospitals, clinics, etc. Fines will be large if the mandates are ignored and mass education and government ads will warn all of pesticide dangers.

PART THREE
What's Happening
To Our Little Girls?

Julianne is a clinical nutritionist and a devoted mother of a beautiful and vivacious daughter, Sarah. But all was not as it seemed. At five years of age, Sarah's breasts began developing. Julianne tells the story of her daughter's experience with early puberty.

One August night in 1999, my daughter, Sarah, who was almost five years old at the time, was about to go to bed. We were going through our normal bedtime routine, when I pulled her pajama top down over her head, suddenly, she yelled "Ouch! That hurt when you touched me. "Surprised by her response, I asked her to show me where it hurt. She lifted up her pajama top, touched her nipples. "It hurt when you put my top over these."

I hadn't really taken a long hard look at her nipples for some time. Now, when I looked closer, they did appear to be different from what I had remembered. In fact, they looked bigger. Then I asked Sarah if her nipples hurt every time I touch them. "Yes," she replied. I continued to question her about how long her nipples had been feeling sore? I was unprepared for her answer. "As long as I can remember."

Her comment came as a complete surprise since she had never mentioned this before. I examined her breast area gently feeling for any irregularities. Everything seemed normal except the area directly below the nipples. My fingers found small lumps there. Not wanting to raise alarm, I assured Sarah everything was perfectly OK, gave her a goodnight kiss and closed the bedroom door.

On the other side of the door, my emotions were racing between shock, fear and panic.

The very first thing I did the next morning was to call my pediatrician. He scheduled an appointment immediately. After examining Sarah, he believed she had some state of premature breast development happening. He referred me on to an endocrinologist.

A month later the endocrinologist ran a series of hormone tests to check Sarah's estrogen and pituitary hormone levels. This condition is considered an abnormality of the pituitary gland.

The results of the test confirmed that Sarah was going through puberty. The small lumps were breast buds. Sarah's breasts were actually developing. But she was only five years old!! How could this possible be? The doctor explained Sarah had a condition called " ". While still a highly unusual situation, she said it was happening with more frequency.

I sat there in shock as the specialist went on to inform me the medical community now considers eight years of age to the be normal age for the beginning of puberty! Previously it was twelve. While I always believed little girls go through puberty at around eleven, twelve or thirteen years of age, something very strange was now happening to our daughters. I was now being told little girls are considered "normal" if they start menstruating at the delicate age of eight!

But there is nothing normal about a five years old racing headlong into puberty.

Because precocious puberty is now a medical reality, there are books written to help children understand what's happening to their bodies. My doctor's office provides copies of "The Story of Tommy Too -Soon". Which tries to explain to these children about the changes going on in their bodies are a "too soon" problem. Trying to explain puberty, and all that it means to five year old, would be much too difficult.

After considering the options, the doctor's recommendation was monthly injections of a hormone-blocking drug called Lupron. It is the only recognized treatment for precocious puberty blocking the release of gonadatropin-releasing hormone made by the pituitary gland. Lupron is normally used for the treatment of prostate cancer in older men. Pediatric medicine has also begun using it to treat precocious puberty.

I was most concerned about using this drug. After all, it hadn't been used very long for precocious puberty. What health problems might be expected? The doctor was recommending monthly injections until Sarah was eleven years old – that was six years of monthly shots! The doctor did his best to reassure me. However, from my own research about Lupron, I learned there were, in fact, many side effects (according to the Physicians' Desk Reference, Lupron has 265 possible side effects). I wasn't at all certain about the use of Lupron in children since it was only approved for pediatric use in the mid 1980's. There are no long-term studies. Understandably, I was really worried.

However, after extensive research, I realized there just weren't any other alternative treatments successfully blocking the pituitary hormones. If the hormonal surges of puberty signal the bones to stop growing and developing were allowed to continue then Sarah would become a dwarf. Feeling I had no other choice I agreed.

Sarah began monthly injections of Lupron. Thank God for insurance since the shots are very expensive. They cost between $550 - $800 per shot, and they are also quite painful. Lupron is administered intramuscularly in the buttocks with a big needle. To help ease her pain a topical anesthetic was once recommended. Sarah didn't tolerate it very well and it didn't really numb the area anyway, so we discontinued using it. During every visit, her father and I have to literally hold her down. Needless to say, this monthly visit is extremely stressful for all of us, including the nursing staff.

I often think about what could have caused this to happen. I wasn't able to breast feed due to a very complicated delivery. Therefore, I fed her formula. Unfortunately there aren't any organic formulas on the market. My real suspicion has to due with estrogenic influences in the formula and diet from the endocrine-disrupting compounds contaminating the food supply. As a nutritionist, I had made sure Sarah ate the healthiest diet. I believe that her soy formula had something to due with her condition. Sarah loved it so much she used to drink a big cup of it every night right up to five years of age. Of course, I stopped the formula right after her diagnosis. We are now two years down the track and Sarah seems to be tolerating the treatments well. This has become a medical reality in our family and one that we have come to live with. However, we still don't know what the long-term outcome will be for our daughter.

These days, it's certainly a challenge keeping little girls, as little girls. The teenybopper fascination with such sexy symbols as Britney Spears has little girls trying to act much older than they are. If bearing the belly button in sexy midriff tops doesn't cause great consternation to parents, the growing phenomenon of budding breasts and pubic hair certainly does. Discovering your little girl has breast buds or pubic hair is a shock to parents for which they are totally unprepared.

Early sexual development in girls, known as precocious puberty, seems to be happening everywhere. Just look around at little girls these days. On the playground you can spot the 9 and 10-year-old girls with developing breasts. Third grade girls look like they belong in middle school while middle schoolers are being mistaken as high school students. Something is seriously amiss.

The onset of menstruation has been steadily declining in Western countries. It wasn't so long ago when a girl's first period ocurred when she was fourteen or fifteen. Today the average age of the first menstruation for causasian girls is 12.8 years. For Afro-Americans, it's currently about six months earlier.

A groundbreaking study in 1997 by Marcia Herman-Giddens, adjunct professor at the University of North Carolina School of Public Health on 17,000 girls, sent shock waves through the medical community. The study that was published in the journal *Pediatrics* found the initial signs of puberty were occurring earlier than previously recorded. The study found 27 percent of African-American and almost 7 percent of causasian girls had the onset of secondary sexual characteristic i.e., either breast development or pubic hair developments by age seven. By the time girls turn eight years old, one in seven caucasian girls and one out of two African-American girls will be starting puberty! Even more startling was the finding that 1 percent of caucasian and 3 percent of African-American girls show these characteristics by the age of three![1]

How common is this trend? "Everyday we encounter young girls, in the 5 to 10 year old range with breasts and pubic hair in our clinic," says Michael Feemark, chief of pediatric endocrinology at Duke University Medical Center in Durham, North Carolina.[2]

The development of secondary sexual characteristics in girls is a significant event, signaling the onset of physiological and psychological ranges of profound importance. Many scientist and doctors are worried. "What we're seeing here is a symptom of a very serious public health problem," says Herman-Giddens.[3] Before they have outgrown dollhouses, many young girls are being faced with the confusing moods swings, hormonal changes and sexual attention accompanying physical maturation.

The problem isn't confined to just the United States. It is a worrying pattern emerging to young girls all over the world. Reports of early puberty have come from many diverse countries and climates including Australia, Canada, England, Europe, Asia and the Caribbean. For instance, the Shanghai Children's Medical Studies Centre alone has reported precocious puberty cases make up nearly half of the 300 to 400 patients who visit the center every month.

Precocious puberty presents dramatic public health problems. Studies have found girls who reach puberty earlier tend to have sex earlier, experience more psychological stress, poorer mental health, more behavioral problems, drink alcohol more often, smoke, have a lower IQ and are at greater risk of committing suicide.

Boys and Early Sexual Development

Early sexual development is not a phenomena occurring only in girls. Boys are also experiencing their version of precocious puberty. Research published in the journal *Archives of Pediatric and Adolescent Medicine* found that American boys appear to be beginning puberty earlier than in past decades. A significant number of boys as young as eight had signs of genital development some three years earlier than previous estimates.[4] In the UK, it is estimated that one in 14 eight-year-old British boys had pubic hair, in contrast to one in 150 boys of the previous generation

Boys as young as nine years old are developing mature genitalia, producing sperm, and have spontaneous erections. In addition, they have hair growth on the face, under arms and in the pubic area along with acne problems. With surging testosterone levels, they are also preoccupied with girls.

The health risk of early puberty in males includes an increased incidence of testicular cancer, lower fertility rates and impaired growth leading to a shorter stature.

Early Puberty and Breast Cancer Risk

But the most disturbing consequence of early puberty in girls is the well-established risk for pre and postmenopausal breast cancer as well as ovarian cancer. According to a study published in 1989 in the magazine, *Nature*, the risk associated with having signs of early menarche (onset of menstruation), for instance, one that takes place at the age of 10, is approximately twice that associated with menarche occurring much later, say at the age of 16 or so.[5] In addition, girls showing early sign of puberty also have increased risks of infertility.

A recent study of twins also suggests early puberty may trigger breast cancer in women who are already at unusually high risk due to their genetic makeup. However, the new study suggests going through puberty early may be especially ominous for some women.

For women genetically predisposed to the disease, the rush

of hormones at puberty alone, rather than long-term exposure, may result in breast cancer later in life.

The study looked at 1,811 sets of identical and fraternal female twins. In each set, one or both twins had breast cancer. One thing stood out. For identical twins with cancer, the first twin to reach puberty was five times as likely to get the disease first. The link was even stronger when menstruation began early, before the age of 12. Other factors, a later age at menopause, fewer children and a later first pregnancy, made no difference.

JoAnn Manson of Harvard's Brigham and Women's Hospital said the implications of the study are worrisome given the gradual decline in the age of puberty in the U.S. and the rise in childhood obesity. Body fat can stimulate hormones. If the findings are correct, "There's even more impetus to try to reverse this epidemic of obesity in children."[6]

Since early puberty is a well-established risk for breast cancer, the earlier a woman reaches puberty, the longer her breast tissues will be exposed to potentially harmful-causing agents (chemicals, radiation, and estrogen). Early puberty, combined with having children later, or not having them at all, is yet another factor increasing a woman's susceptibility.

"The length and amount of exposure to estrogen is one of the most significant risk factors in breast carcinogenesis. Unless you are exposed to estrogens, you don't get breast cancer. The longer the exposure is, the higher the incidence. Therefore if you decrease the age of menarche (first menstruation), you are at higher risk," warns Carlos Sonnenschein of the Tufts University of Medicine in Boston.[7]

The Obesity Connection

The experts are confused. Some scientists think early puberty is due to improved nutrition, a rather questionable premise considering the appalling state of the typical Western diet.

However, other causes are much more plausible. The front-runner appears to be related to an increase in obesity in children. In the United States and Canada, more than one third of children between the ages of 2 and 11 are overweight. One half of them are considered obese. Overweight girls also have more insulin circulating in their blood. Why is that a problem? Higher insulin levels appear to stimulate the production of sex hormones from the ovaries and adrenal glands.

Early breast development seems to be encouraged by a recently discovered hormone called leptin. Leptin is necessary for the progression of puberty. Obese people have high leptin levels circulating in their blood. Leptin links puberty to obesity because leptin is produced from fat cells. More adipose tissue leads to more leptin, which is a trigger for earlier puberty.

Could prenatal exposure to endocrine disrupters play a role in obesity? Animal studies have given us important clues. Puberty can be advanced experimentally in mice by increasing leptin levels. Data from animals suggests contamination from hormone disrupting chemicals may also be involved by interfering with leptin's role in weight regulation.[8]

The Hormone Disrupting Chemical Connection

Experiments with animals demonstrate conclusively the pace and pattern of sexual development is vulnerable to chemical contamination either while the womb or shortly after birth.

One significant study found that when female mice were fed food containing low doses of bisphenol A, their female offspring began sexual development significantly earlier than the unexposed mice.[9]

Is this also true for humans? It seems so. A twenty-year study followed 302 girls and 267 boys who had been exposed to PCBs. The researchers found the higher the level of prenatal PCB exposure, the heavier the girls were at age 14 and their puberty was statistically earlier.[10]

In fact, the really guilty party is looking more and more like environmental endocrine disrupters.

An important part of unraveling this puzzle came from studies in Puerto Rico. As was discussed earlier, for the past two decades, Puerto Rico has had the highest known incidence of premature breast development, known as thelarche ever reported. Girls, as young as two years of age, were showing signs of breast development.

Although soy formulas have been considered one of the culprits, more clues are emerging implicating endocrine disruptors as well. The early breast development was linked to phthalate exposure. Researchers measured the presence of certain phthalates in the blood of girls experiencing early breast development. The average age of these girls was 31 months.

The phthalates found in the thelarche group are known to have estrogenic and anti-androgenic effects. Anti-androgenic means "interferes with male hormone." Humans of both genders always have a mix of male and female hormones in their blood stream, the balance between them being important.[11]

Phthalates are now everywhere. They are common industrial chemicals used in building materials, food packaging and food wrap, toys and other children's products, medical devices, garden hose, shoes, shoe soles, automobile undercoating, wires and cables, carpet backing, carpet tile, vinyl tile, pool liners, artificial leather, canvas tarps, notebook covers, tool handles, dishwasher baskets, flea collars, insect repellents, skin emollients, hair sprays, nail polish, and perfumes, among other uses.

A study measuring the metabolic byproducts of 7 phthalates found them in the urine of the adult subjects. The researchers concluded exposure to phthalates "is both higher and more common than previously suspected." The highest levels (1 to 16 parts per million in urine) were phthalates occurring at the highest levels in women of childbearing age.[12]

They also found a high levels of a chemical called DEPH, a

known anti-androgen. Girls with premature breast development showed DEPH concentrations almost 7 times higher than the control group. Unfortunately, the sparseness of the scientific literature indicates most compounds have not been tested. However, the studies that have been done reveal very strong effects, suggesting other hormonally-active compounds, not yet studied, will also have impacts.

Mounting Evidence

The biological clock also seems to be speeding up for the daughters of women accidentally exposed to a fire retardant chemical, polybrominated biphenyl, or PBB, nearly three decades ago. Early puberty is much more common among these young women. A new study suggests the change may be linked to their mothers' contact with PBB.

In 1973, several thousand pounds of PBB was accidentally mixed with livestock feed and distributed to farms in Michigan. Over a million chickens, cows, pigs and sheep were contaminated. The problem was only identified when calves were stillborn or born with hoof deformities. This was the largest food contamination incident in American history.

By then, at least 4,000 people had been exposed to the chemical through meat and dairy products. PBB accumulates in fatty tissues around the body and can maintain its presence in people for roughly 13 to 29 years depending on the level of exposure.

Researchers suspected the chemical might interfere with hormone function based on animal studies, so they decided to check out the generation following those exposed in 1973. They contacted all of the female children, born to women exposed to the chemical in the Michigan incident.

They found the mothers with the highest levels of PBB in

their blood, who also breast fed their daughters, produced girls with the earliest menstruation. Girls who received both in utero and breast milk chemical exposure started their periods at the average age of 11.6, a full year earlier than other girls who were not exposed.

Little is known about exactly how PBBs might affect the onset of puberty, although experts say the chemical binds to estrogen receptors and PBBs and polychlorinated biphenyls (PCBs) affect the thyroid gland.

What is coming to light is contaminants can both speed and slow the rate of sexual development. In general, it would appear estrogen mimics increase sexual development in females, while androgen mimics increase the onset of puberty in males. On the other hand, anti-androgens can produce the opposite effect of slowing down sexual development in males.

There's no doubt about it. Endocrine disruptors are affecting both little girls and little boys.

Commercially grown meat and dairy consistently have the highest levels of persistent hormone disruptors.

As of 1995, the FDA allowed the use of implanted hormonal agents for raising beef cattle. These include the female hormones estradiol and progesterone, norgestomet, synthetic progesterone, the male hormone testosterone and the synthetic anabolic steroid zeranol and trenbolene. Growth agents do not have to be implanted. A progestin can be added to the animals' feed. None of the hormonal agents require a withdrawal period prior to slaughter. In fact, the FDA does not require mandatory recording of medication or treatment of meat animals.

Hormones in beef have serious estrogenic and carcinogenic effects - effects of which the cancer establishment, the FDA, and the cattle industry have been well aware for decades. Yet the real dangers they pose, especially when it comes to women and breast cancer, have remained in the shadows until the present. (Pork, veal, lamb poultry and other cuts of meat, although uncontaminated by sex hormones, contain pesticides and a wide range of veterinary drugs.)[1]

Not surprisingly, a random survey in 1986 found up to half of all cattle sampled in feedlots in Kansas, Colorado, Texas, Nebraska and Oklahoma had hormone pellets illegally implanted in muscle tissue rather than under the ear. This practice led to higher absorption of hormones from the implants and very much higher residues which the FDA admitted could have "adverse effects".[2]

According to Samuel S. Epstein, M.D. Professor Emeritus of Environmental and Occupational Medicine at the University of Illinois School of Public Health and Chairman of the Cancer Prevention Coalition, "Records of hormone levels in beef obtained under the Federal Freedom of Information Act from the FDA, show when ranchers implant single hormone pellets beneath the ear skin under ideal laboratory conditions, levels of estradiol and other hormones in meat and organs are more than triple the levels found in non- implanted controls. Much higher levels, up to three-hundred-fold, result from the common practice of illegal intramuscular implants."[3]

The US Department of Agriculture inspectors have reported finding the pellets in the crown of the head, between the ears, behind the neck, at the base of the ear, and chest area of cattle carcasses.

Cattle today are receiving a lot more hormones than ever before. In 1990, the FDA ruled in favor of doubling the dose of hormones allowed in cattle. As a result of this new ruling, some feedlots now put implants in each ear for more bulk at a faster rate. This is because feedlots are paid by weight for their product.

The FDA's reports in hormonal implants give us cause to worry. In 1983, the FDA found that Synovex-S, a product containing estradiol and progestin, increased estradiol concentrations in cattle muscle by twelve-fold, in liver by six-fold, in kidneys by nine-fold and in fat by twenty-threefold. When cattle are slaughtered following implantation, levels are ever higher. With multiple implants, they are higher still; with intramuscular implants, yet even higher. Some hormones are also added to the cattle's feed in feedlots.

The extent to which hormonally laden meat contributes to increased breast cancer rates, apart from cancer of the uterus, prostate and testes, has been virtually ignored. Hormonal beef may also have other endocrine-disruptive effects including initiating early puberty.

Is comes as no surprise the European Union has banned hormone-treated US beef. Americans unfortunately, are getting a pharmacopoeia of steroid drugs every time they chow down a hamburger or hot dog. For children, eating hormone-laced meat on a regular basis seriously increases their estrogen exposure.

Animals Raised the Way Nature Intended

It should be obvious by now, organically raised meat is the only safe meat to eat. Meat should be free of chemicals, sprayed feed, antibiotics and hormone injected growth stimulators. Organic, grass-fed beef is by far healthier and more nutritious than the commercial kind. Grass-fed beef means cattle being fed on natural grass pasture their entire life rather than "finished off" on corn or soy meal. Corn and soy are unnatural foods for cattle causing an overly acidic condition resulting in more health problems.

Grass-fed beef have high levels of key nutrients. For example, grass-fed products are rich in all the fats now proven to be health-enhancing, such as omega 3's but low in the fats linked with disease like too much omega 6's. The meat and milk from grass-fed cows are the richest known source of another good fat called "conjugated linoleic acid" or CLA. When ruminants are raised on fresh pasture alone, their milk and meat contain as much as five times more CLA than products from animals fed conventional diets.

CLA may be one of our most potent defenses against cancer. In laboratory animals, a very small percentage of CLA (a mere 0.1 percent of total calories) greatly reduces tumor growths. Grass-fed beef is also full of other key nutrients like beta-carotene and have over 400 percent more vitamins A and E.

What about poultry and fish? Growth promoters and antibiotics are widely used in the commercial poultry industry. Organic chickens and turkey are, without doubt, the safest. Fish has always been considered a healthy alternative to meat. Unfortunately, it is getting more and more difficult to find clean fish, either fresh water or ocean. Fresh water fish appear to be among the most heavily contaminated of foods. Top predator fish, like pike and walleye are likely to be contaminated with heavy metal, mercury, other known hormone disruptors. Shellfish often concentrate cadmium, another endocrine-disrupting heavy metal. Diets high in adequate calcium, protein, iron and zinc help protect against cadmium absorption. The very best fish to eat are deep-sea fish such as halibut, Alaskan salmon, sardines, cod and mackerel.

Americans love their dairy. In 1970, the average American ate ten pounds of cheese. In the year 2000, the average American ate over thirty pounds of cheese. Since it takes ten pounds of milk to manufacture one pound of hard cheese, the average American is exposed to three hundred pounds of milk, concentrated into those thirty pounds. Every sip of cow's milk contains estrogen, progesterone, prolactin, melatonin, and other female steroid hormones.[11] Those hormones are only the naturally occurring ones, not the synthetic ones.

D. Lindsey Berkson, author of *Hormone Deception*, issues strong warnings about milk and milk products:

> Milk and milk products are a sacred cow in the United States, perhaps due to the fact that the United Dairy Industry Association spends more than $100 million a year on advertising, targeting women. Good consumers that we are, we proudly wear our milk moustaches. Along with the milk, we unwittingly swallow bovine growth hormone (BGH), an estrogenic hormone given to cows. BGH may be good for dairy farmers because it increases milk production, but it may not be good for humans. Why? Because BGH has been implicated in the increased risk of breast cancer.
>
> BGH also contributes to the hormone disruptor soup through another route. Although the FDA approved the drug, it admits the use of this growth hormone often causes udder infections in cows. This leads to puss and bacteria getting into the milk. To prevent this, cows on BGH are given more antibiotics. Certain subclasses of antibiotics, are themselves, estrogenic or hormone disruptors."[1]

Recent studies in the prestigious *International Journal of Health Sciences* concludes super-charged levels of Insulin Growth Factor - 1, a hormone which regulates cell division and growth, found in dairy products from treated cows are likely to pose risks of breast cancer by stimulating cell division and prompting malignant transformation of normal breast cells. At greater risk are infants and children, who traditionally drink a lot of milk.

The Raw Milk Comeback

Do we need to abandon our milk passions? No, not at all! While modern milk production has seriously altered what once was a most healthy and nutritious food, there is a growing resurgence in the benefits of raw, unpasteurized milk and milk products.

It's wasn't' that long ago when raw milk was the only way to get milk and its benefits. However, when modern milk processing came into vogue, along with less sanitary conditions, raw milk and raw milk products all but disappeared. The acceptance of homogenized and pasteurized milk was accompanied by a huge increase in many health problems for both children and adults.

Research on children showed children fed raw milk have more resistance to TB, scurvy, flu, diphtheria, pneumonia, asthma, allergic skin problems and tooth decay. In addition, their growth and calcium absorption was superior.

Raw milk has many health benefits. It contains all 22 amino acids. Pasteurized milk, on the other hand, severely alters the amino acids, making them less available to your body. Raw milk has trace minerals as well as 100 per cent of the minerals metabolically available to your body (calcium, chlorine, magnesium, phosphorus, potassium, sodium, and sulphur).

Pasteurization alters calcium leaving 50 percent or less of it able to be absorbed by your body. Other minerals are also less available, as well as the loss of the enzymes serving as catalysts for the assimilation of minerals into the body. Another benefit of raw milk is that all fat soluble and water soluble vitamins are 100 percent metabolically available while pasteurized milk has up to a 66 percent loss of vitamins A, D, E, and F; more than a 50 percent loss of vitamin C; a loss of 38– 80 percent of all water soluble vitamins; and the complete destruction of the vitamins B-6 and B-12.

Both raw and pasteurized milk harbor bacteria but the bacteria in raw milk is the healthy bacteria of lactic acid fermentation while the bacteria in pasteurized milk is the bacteria of spoilage. Additionally overall bacteria count of milk produced under clean conditions is much lower than pasteurized milk.

While homogenized and pasteurized cow's milk poses a serious threat to the health and well-being of children (and adults), goat's milk is another milk choice that comes to the rescue. Goat's milk most imitates human milk in composition. It is praised because it is readily digestible. Goat's milk is digested in just 20 minutes while cow's milk takes between two to three hours.

One of goat's milk secrets lies in its natural ability to be half cleansing and half building. It contains a unique balance of vitamins, minerals, proteins, carbohydrates, enzymes and fats. It is one of the few whole foods actually able to sustain life. Goat's milk assists in the healing of a wide variety of disorders including ulcers, arthritis, rheumatism, irritable bowel syndrome, Crohn's disease, fibromyalgia, leaky gut syndrome, anxiety disorders, anorexia, asthma, and food allergies. The high nutritional quality and the greater ease of digestion are what make goat's milk so effective. Needless to say, organic and unpasteurized is always best.

Over the last several decades about 80 percent of the food supply has been processed by the food industry. The additives used are increasing at a rate of 4 to 5 percent annually. One such additive is a carcinogenic food coloring called Red Dye No. 3 which the food industry uses to color bubble gum, maraschino cherries, strawberry milk shakes and a wide range of snack foods and baked products.

A 1997 report in *Environment Health Perspective* estimated the diet of Americans is increasingly made of processed foods likely to contain food colorants such as Red Dye No. 3. These colorants bind to estrogen receptors on breast cells and derange the cells' DNA. Exposure to this synthetic dye increases the risk of cancer, especially breast cancer.[1] Researchers estimate the average woman receives a daily dose of Red Dye No. 3 about 1000 to 2000 times the amount required to derange the DNA of cells. Imagine how this level of exposure is wreaking havoc in our children who are ingesting these chemicals day in and day out.

In 1990 the FDA discontinued the use of a form of Red Dye No. 3 which was used to make external drugs and cosmetics because of reports the chemical caused thyroid cancers in rats. However, it is still allowed to be used as a food "dye". Since this ingredient and other food additives are rarely, if ever, listed as ingredients, the unsuspecting public has no idea of what is hiding in each swallow or slurp.

Most of our supermarket foods contain a variety of food additives and dyes. The FDA, however, does not require flavor companies to disclose the ingredients of their additives as long as all the chemicals are considered by the agency to be GRAS (Generally Regarded as Safe). This lack of public disclosure enables the companies to maintain the secrecy of their formulas. It also hides the facts when flavor compounds contain more ingredients than the foods which are being flavored. The most dangerous and least necessary additives are dyes.

Dyes are a trap for the unwary, especially children who are attracted to the bright shiny colors. Dyes are derived from coal tar, a known carcinogen. Tartrazine, for example, is used to dye food yellow, orange, and green and is found in sodas, jams, decorations, custard, flavored milk and many bakery goods. Approximately 10 percent of the public is intolerant or allergic to it. It is also linked to cancer of the intestinal tract, skin and respiratory problems and is considered a central nervous system poison.

The ubiquitous phrase "artificial strawberry flavor" gives little hint of the chemical wizardry making highly process food taste like strawberry. For instance, a typical artificial strawberry flavor contains the following ingredients:

amyl acetate, amyl butyrate, amyl valerate, anethol, anisyl formate, benyl acetate, benzyl isobutyrate, butyric acid, cinnamyl isobutyrate, cinnamyl valerate, cognac essential oil, diacetyl, dipropyl ketone ethyl butyrate, ethyl cinnamate, ethyl heptanoate, ethyl heptylate, ethyl lactate, ethyl methylphenylglycidate, ethyl nitrate, ethyl propionaaate, ethyl valerate, heliotropin, hydoxyphrenyl-2-butanone, a-ionone, isobutyl anthranilate, isobutyl butyrate, lemon essential oil, maltol, 4-methyl-cetphenone, methyl anthranilate, methyl benzoate, methyl cinnamate, methyl heptine carbonate, methyl naphthhyl ketone, methyl salicylate, mint essential oil, neroli essential oil, neryl isobutyrate, orris butter, phenethyl alcohol, rose, rum ether, y-undecalactone, vanillin and solvent.[3]

That's over 40 different chemicals and not a trace of real strawberry to be found anywhere.

So the next time you eat some strawberry ice cream, strawberry topping, or anything tasting like or looking like strawberry, what you're most likely savoring is the chemical miracle of modern food science. It's impossible to even guess what the consequences of all those chemicals on a young person's body. I have only listed the chemical soup for just one kind of flavoring. What about dozens of other artificial "natural" flavors permeating hundreds, if not thousands, of products lining our supermarket shelves.

It's not only what we eat, but also what we eat out of that contains hormone disruptors. Packaging materials, such as styrene cups, trays for microwaving prepared foods, cling wrap, and the lining of canned foods, also contain estrogenic chemicals. Alkyphenols, nonylphenol and bisphenol A, all which are used in food packaging materials and all known hormone disruptors, migrate into foods, particularly when stored for long periods or heated at high temperatures.

Americans have a mighty hankering for sugar. It seems we just can't get enough of the stuff. On average, a half a cup of sugar is consumed per-person every day. It is estimated the average American eats, drinks, slurps, stirs, and sprinkles about 150 pounds of it annually. Other Western countries fall right in line. Never in modern history has a culture consumed so much sugar.

There is probably no other ingredient more ubiquitous or goes by so many names than sugar. What we call sugar— whether white, granulated, or table—is one type of sugar called sucrose and is only the tip of the crystal. Maltose, more commonly called malt sugar, is present in beer and works the quickest. Glucose, the primary sugar in corn syrup, is not far behind, and dextrose is the same as glucose. Sucrose, processed from sugar cane or sugar beets, has the next quickest effect. It includes brown sugar, turbinate sugar, and the sugar in molasses. There are actually more than 100 different sucrose substances.

It truly does deserve its reputation as a 'white poison'. Thinking of sugar as a food is really a stretch of the imagination since it is more like a chemical and is difficult for the body to utilize and digest. Humans were really not designed to eat large amounts of sugar in whatever form it may take - white and brown, corn syrup, sucrose, dextrose, glucose, fructose, lactose, maltose, barley malt, honey, rice syrup and maple syrup. Sugar is also highly seductive, acting as an addictive-like drug luring even the most well-intentioned person back into its sweet clutches.

Sugar leaches the body of vital minerals and vitamins. It raises blood pressure, triglycerides and the bad cholesterol (LDL) increasing the risk of heart disease. It causes tooth decay and periodontal disease which leads to tooth loss and systemic infections. It makes it difficult for a child's brain to learn resulting in a lack of concentration. Sugar consumption causes both children and adults to exhibit disruptive behavior, learning disorder, and forgetfulness. It initiates autoimmune and immune deficiency disorders such as arthritis, allergies and asthma. It also upsets hormonal balance and supports the growth of cancer cells. Sugar can cause hypoglycaemia and weight gain leading to diabetes and obesity both in children and adults.

Breast cancer susceptibility can be increased if soft drinks are consumed on a regular basis. After drinking soft drinks, there is a fast and dramatic increase in both glucose and insulin levels within the first hour. This response is more pronounced in children. Increased insulin leads to higher circulating Insulin Growth Factor-1 which increases breast cancer risk sevenfold. Therefore, girls who consume soft drinks regularly increase their breast cancer risk later in life.[1]

Teenage girls consume about 12 ounces of soda a day. Each can of soda contains about 10 teaspoons of sugar. Coke, Pepsi, Mountain Dew and Dr. Pepper also contain caffeine. Soft drink consumption has also become commonplace among toddlers. About one-fifth of America's one and two-year olds now regularly drink soda. In a 1999 study by the Center for Science in the Public Interest called "Liquid Candy" "Pepsi, Dr. Pepper and Seven-Up encourage feeding soft drinks to babies by licensing their logos to a major maker of baby bottles, Munchkin Bottling, Inc. A 1997 study published in the *Journal of Dentistry for Children* found many infants were indeed being fed soda in those bottles.[2]

Sugar should be avoided as much as possible. But don't think switching over to diet drinks with Nutrasweet or artificial sweeteners will get you out of the woods. Far from it, you will still be in the deepest part of the forest.

Aspartame: Not so Sweet

If sugar is out, then the sugar substitute Aspartame must be in, right? Wrong!

Millions of people use aspartame, the artificial sweetener known as NutraSweet™. However, aspartame's tainted history of approval and potentially toxic ingredients cast a serious doubt on the safety of this sugar substitute. Furthermore, even though aspartame is marketed as a low-calorie sweetener, it actually increases one's appetite! While FDA approval may signal the green light for safe consumption, 85 percent of all complaints registered with the FDA are for adverse reactions to aspartame. A closer look at the unscientific studies, suspicious approval methods, and its harmful ingredients, reveal the hidden dangers of this artificial sweetener. In reality, aspartame poses an urgent public health threat.

Many of these reactions are very serious including seizures and death. A few of the 90 different documented symptoms listed in the report being caused by aspartame include: headaches, migraines, dizziness, seizures, nausea, numbness, muscle spasms, weight gain, rashes, depression, fatigue, irritability, tachycardia, insomnia, vision problems, hearing loss, heart palpitations, breathing difficulties, anxiety attacks, slurred speech, loss of taste, tinnitus, vertigo, memory loss, and joint pain.

According to researchers and physicians studying the adverse effects of aspartame, the following chronic illnesses can be triggered or worsened by ingesting of aspartame: brain tumors, multiple sclerosis, epilepsy, chronic fatigue syndrome, Parkinson's disease, Alzheimer's, mental retardation, lymphoma, birth defects, fibromyalgia, and diabetes.

Dr. George Schwartz, a medical doctor, researcher and author wrote the following in the *Western Journal of Medicine*, "I discovered an extraordinary correlation between aspartame (marketed as NutraSweet and in its generic form) and increasing breast and prostate cancer incidence."[3]

Interestingly, breast and prostate cancer rates are 5 to 6 times higher in Europe and North America than in Asia and Africa, the latter correlating with lower use of NutraSweet.[4,5]

Also, a review of the original NutraSweet animal laboratory research findings, released under the Freedom of Information Act, revealed mammary tumors were observed in many of the test animals.

The correlation associated with aspartame consumption and cancer in susceptible people points to a need for immediate scrutiny of aspartame as an environmental cause of many thousands of cancer cases.

Ok, so aspartame is not the answer. What about the new miracle sweetener, sucrolose, sold under the brand name Splenda which is non-caloric and about 600 times sweeter than white sugar. Aside from the fact there are no long term studies ensuring its safety, research in animals has shown sucrolose has caused many problems. Some of the side-effects include: shrunken thymus glands (up to 40 percent shrinkage), enlarged liver and kidneys, reduced growth rate, decreased body weights and placental weights.

Although sucrolose is finding its way into many foods, even those marketed as healthy and sold in health food stores, it should certainly be avoided, especially by children.

Deadly Sweet - The 25 Top Reasons to Avoid Sugar

In addition to throwing off the body's homeostasis, excess sugar may result in a number of other significant consequences. The following is a listing of some of sugar's metabolic consequences from a variety of medical journals and other scientific publications.

1. Sugar can suppress the immune system.
2. Sugar can upset the body's mineral balance.
3. Sugar can cause hyperactivity, anxiety, concentration difficulties and crankiness in children.
4. Sugar can cause drowsiness and decreased activity in children.

5. Sugar can adversely affect children's school grades.
6. Sugar contributes to a weakened defense against bacterial infection.
7. Sugar may lead to chromium deficiency.
8. Sugar interferes with absorption of calcium and magnesium.
9. Sugar may lead to cancer of the breast, ovaries, prostate and rectum.
10. Sugar can weaken eyesight.
11. Sugar can cause hypoglycemia.
12. Sugar can raise adrenaline levels in children.
13. Sugar can promote tooth decay.
14. Sugar can contribute to weight gain and obesity.
15. Sugar increases the risk of Crohn's disease and ulcerative colitis.
16. Sugar can cause asthma.
17. Sugar can cause candidiasis (yeast infection).
18. Sugar can cause appendicitis.
19. Sugar can lead to periodontal disease.
20. Sugar causes food allergies.
21. Sugar can contribute to eczema in children.
22. Sugar can cause myopia (nearsightedness).
23. Sugar can cause headaches, including migraines.
24. Sugar can cause depression.
25. Sugar can cause hormonal imbalance.

The Three Musketeers of Healthy Sweeteners
Stevia, Lo Han and Xylitol

All is not lost in the world of sugary goodness. Sweetness is a fundamental flavor. In fact, according to Chinese medicine, is absolutely necessary to health. Of course, moderation is the key along with the right kind of sweetness. It's a good idea to limit sugary treats to once a week.

However, before everyone starts singing the sugar blues, there actually are three exciting sweeteners that have all of sugar's sweetness but none of its faults. The 3 musketeers of healthy sweeteners are Stevia, Lo Han and Xylitol.

Stevia - The Gift from South America

If you were to journey into the jungles of Paraguay, you would discover the indigenous Indians chewing the green leaves from a small shrub. For centuries these peoples knew the healing properties of this very sweet leaf from the stevia plant.

Stevia is a popular sweetener because it is – 300 times sweeter than sugar. Its sweetness makes it an appealing alternative to sugar. It has a long history of safe and therapeutic use as an herbal sweetener. The good news is that it has no calories, is zero on the glycemic index and is heat stable making it ideal for cooking and baking. It also enhances the flavor of whatever it's used for. As an extra bonus, stevia helps balance the pancreas which is essential for digestive health.

Stevia's beneficial effect in balancing blood sugar has made it a useful herbal remedy for diabetes and hypoglycemia. Another wonderful quality is its ability to inhibit sugar cravings. The smallest amount will provide the sweetness that most people require – a pinch of stevia has the same impact as a cup of sugar.

It's not only for its sweetness stevia is sought after. Stevia also has many medicinal properties. It is an antifungal, anti-inflammatory and antibiotic agent. Another beneficial property of stevia is its tendency to lower elevated blood pressure while not affecting people with normal blood pressure.

Unlike most sugars, stevia also inhibits the growth and reproduction of oral bacteria and other infectious organisms. Regular users of stevia as a mouthwash or for brushing teeth (added to toothpaste) have improved bleeding gums. This inhibition of oral bacteria may explain why stevia-enhanced products help lower the incidence of colds and flu.

Studies have shown stevia as an exceptional aid in weight loss and weight management because it contains no calories and reduces the craving for sweets and fatty foods. The most important thing to remember when using stevia is not to use too much, or the result is excessive sweetness and a bitter aftertaste. Remember, a little bit goes a long way.

Stevia is delicious in almost any recipe using fruit or dairy products, but does present a bit of a challenge when used for baking, since it lacks sugar's abilities to add texture, help soften batter, caramelize, enhance the browning process, and feed the fermentation of yeast.

When looking for stevia, make sure you buy the best grade possible. Stevia leaves vary widely in quality due to environmental factors including soil, irrigation methods, sunlight, air purity, cleanliness, farming practices, processing and storage. In general, Paraguayan leaves contain 9–13 percent of the sweet molecules steviosides/rebaudiosides, while Chinese stevia contains only 5–6 percent. So the unprocessed Paraguayan stevia will taste better.

Stevia is available either as a powder or a liquid.

Lo Han - An Ancient Plant for Modern Times

Chances are you have never heard of a very special sweetener called Lo Han. This is about to change as the word about Lo Han gets out. Traditionally grown in remote, mountainous areas of southern China, Lo Han has been revered for centuries as a healing fruit.

Lo Han is a small gourd-like fruit of the plant *Momordica grosvenorii* and is in the same family as the cucumber, melon, and squash. Lo Han's active components, like stevia, are approximately 200-300 times as sweet as sucrose. Since Lo Han has been safely used as a food by millions of Chinese, it has been granted GRAS (Generally Recognized As Safe) status, and no restrictions apply to its food use in the U.S.

As an historical herbal remedy, Lo Han extracts have been used for centuries to promote respiratory health and to provide relief of respiratory problems. It is also believed Lo Han helps clear the lungs of airborne pollutants.

Modern scientific experiments show Lo Han fruit extract helps relieve gastritis, constipation, respiratory inflammations, coughs, improves digestion, moisturizes the skin and strengthens the immune system. It also is useful for preventing cavities. The good news is no side effects have ever been documented.

The pulp of the fruit is intensely sweet. Since the body is unable to break down these compounds in the same way it breaks down simple sugars and carbohydrates, it is not metabolized as sugar. Therefore, Lo Han will not promote fat storage nor the insulin, blood sugar and cholesterol surges caused by other forms of sugar. This makes Lo Han a perfect calorie-free and low glycemic sweetener.

Lo Han is especially attractive since it has a very clean taste with no bitter aftertaste. Lo Han is also very stable in the face of heating and freezing, and therefore, can be readily used in cooked/baked goods and in frozen desserts. Lo Han is available in powder form and as a liquid.

Xylitol— Our Sweet Salvation

At the end of World War II, Finland was left in quite a predicament. There was no sugar to be found anywhere. So the Finns searched for an alternative. They found it in the form of xylitol, a natural, low-calorie sugar made from birch bark.

Since then xylitol has been produced from corncobs. Xylitol is a natural substance found in fibrous vegetables, fruits, and in various hardwood trees like birch. It also occurs naturally in our bodies where normal metabolism makes up to 15 grams of the it daily.

Although xylitol tastes and looks exactly like sugar, that is where the similarities end. In fact, xylitol is sugar's mirror image. While sugar wreaks havoc on the body, xylitol, like stevia and lo han, heals and repairs. It also builds immunity, protects against chronic degenerative disease and has anti-aging benefits. Xylitol is an antimicrobial, preventing the growth of bacteria. While sugar is acid forming, xylitol is alkaline enhancing.

Xylitol has 40 percent fewer calories and 75 percent fewer carbohydrates than sugar and is slowly absorbed and metabolized, resulting in negligent changes in insulin levels. In fact, on the glycemic index in which glucose is rated at 100, xylitol weighs in at just 7.

Xylitol has been fully approved by the FDA. The only discomfort some sensitive people may initially notice is a laxative effect occuring only when large amounts are consumed. Since xylitol is naturally made in the body, as well as the enzymes that break it down, any discomfort usually disappears within a few days.

Consistently using small amounts of xylitol tends to increase protective factors in saliva and help maintain an alkaline condition. The oral environment becomes less acidic with continued use of xylitol. It is advised to chew xylitol gum or suck a xylitol mint after every meal or sweet snacks. The best news is that xylitol's effect is long lasting and possibly even permanent.

Another unexpected benefit of xylitol for children, whose teeth are colonized between 19–31 months of age by the bacteria streptococcus mutans are more prone to have a large number of cavities. Most children acquire this bacteria from their mother's saliva from food tasting, sharing cups and kissing. The children whose mothers chewed xylitol gum, showed a 70 percent reduction in tooth decay. Xylitol also successfully eliminates the bacteria that cause sinusitis, throat, ear and lung infections. In addition, it is effective in inhibiting Candida albicans and other harmful gut bacteria.

Reversing bone loss is another exciting benefit from xylitol. Finnish Studies showed that xylitol maintained bone density in rats, with removed ovaries. Without ovaries, estrogen levels plummeted and so did the bone density in the rats not given xylitol. However, in the xylitol-fed rats with removed ovaries, their bone density actually increased. The scientists speculated xylitol's bone density enhancing properties are due to its ability to promote the intestinal absorption of calcium.

Since xylitol is a natural insulin stabilizer, foods sweetened with it will not raise insulin levels. In fact, it actually helps stop sugar and carbohydrate cravings, making it a perfect sweetener for people with diabetes and those wanting to lose weight.

Insulin resistance also plays a significant role in most hormonal imbalances. High insulin levels increase the production of estrogens and interfere with healthy ovarian function. Polycystic ovarian syndrome (PCOS), which can lead to infertility, is a condition becoming more and more common in teenagers and young women. Insulin resistance is a major cause of PCOS. Lowering insulin levels is an effective way of treating PCOS and other hormonal imbalances. Using xylitol instead of sugar (and reducing high glycemic index foods) is a great way to maintain low insulin levels.

Xylitol is the answer to our prayers for satisfying our sweet tooth and be healthy at the same time.

Consumers were recently warned in a report from the Institute of Medicine there is no level of trans fatty acids safe to consume. As a result, many people swung open their pantry doors vowing to purge their lives of trans fats only to find themselves staring into the shelves not really knowing what they were even looking for.

That's because food manufacturers don't have to list the amount of trans fat on the nutrition panel - even though it can be found in more than 40 percent of the food on supermarket shelves.

Trans fat is a processed fat formed by partially hydrogenating edible oil. The result is the fat stays relatively solid at room temperature. Think of trans fat essentially as shortening or margarine. Crisco is a perfect example. It's why your pie crust is so flaky and why Ritz crackers stay crisp. It prolongs shelf life, which is why commercial bakeries love it.

Unfortunately, what is good for commercial bakeries isn't necessarily good for people. The truth is this slick ingredient is a health disaster.

Trans fats cause heart disease and can lead to heart attacks and strokes. The report by the National Academy of Science summarized several studies showing trans fat raises levels of the waxy cholesterol that clogs blood vessels and strips the good kind of cholesterol.

Other studies have connected trans fats to a broader range of health problems, including cancer, insulin resistance, diabetes and increased allergies in children.

Parents may not realize they're feeding the potentially dangerous substance to their babies. Many baby foods contain partially hydrogenated fats. Trans fatty acids replace the essential fatty acids (EFAs) needed for brain growth.

Dr. Walter Willett, Chairman of the Department of Nutrition at the Harvard School of Public Health, is recognized as one of the world's top authorities on nutrition. He calls partial hydrogenation of oils the "biggest food-processing disaster in

U.S. history." He is most concerned about the extent of trans fats found in the American diet. "In Europe [food companies] hired chemists and took out trans fats. In the United States, they hired lawyers and public relations people. No one doubted trans fats have adverse affects on health, and still companies were not taking it out."[1]

So, how much trans fat is considered safe? The National Academies of Sciences report said no level of trans fat is safe. But the researchers recognized it would be impossible to remove trans fats from the American diet, since it's found in more than 40,000 products. Their answer, short of an all-out ban, is to recommend people eat as little as possible.

Here are some things to look for on the label. First, look to see if partially hydrogenated oil is in the ingredient list. How much depends on how high on the list those words appear. Products listing cold/expeller pressed oils, poly or monounsaturated oils, olive oil, coconut oil, palm oil and other liquid oils likely won't have trans fat.

Stay away from partially hydrogenated oils. About 40 percent of products in supermarkets contain them. Some health conscious markets have refused to sell any products containing partially hydrogenated oils.

If the words "partially hydrogenated" or "shortening" are in the list of ingredients, don't buy the product, and if you've already bought it, then throw it away. You can always find an equivalent product just as tasty and without the partially hydrogenated oil.

Watch out! Many products have labels saying they are "trans fat-free" or have "zero grams of trans fat," but they still contain partially hydrogenated oil. That's because under FDA regulations, "if the serving contains less than 0.5 grams, the content, when declared, shall be expressed as zero." It's a very bad rule and should be changed! Some food manufacturers believe this allows them to say on the packaging the product is "trans fat-free."

Sources of trans fats include:

Fast food: Most fast-food and family-style chain restaurants cook fries, chicken and other deep-fried foods in partially hydrogenated oil, which often comes in a solid block melted in the fryer. They also slather margarine - which has trans fats - on griddles for pancakes and grilled sandwiches.

Baked goods: This is the heaviest trans fat territory. Most mass- produced convenience and commercial bakery goods, like cookies and cakes, have plenty of trans fat. Cakes and shortening-based frostings from supermarket bakeries are particularly trans-heavy. So are doughnuts, which can contain shortening in the dough and also be cooked in trans fat. Generally, the higher quality the baked good, the less trans fat, because more butter is used.

Chips and crackers: To keep them crisp, manufacturers pump crackers full of shortening. Even crackers labeled 'reduced fat' can still have trans fat. Watch for anything fried, like potato chips and corn chips, as well as 'buttery' crackers.

Spreads, sauces and mixes: Margarine can be pure trans fat. As a general rule, the softer the margarine, the less artery-clogging fat it contains. There are some trans-fat-free spreads on the market and increasingly are labeled as such. Watch out for high trans-fat levels in non-dairy creamers and flavored coffees, as well as in ready-made dips.

Unexpected places: Breakfast cereals, breakfast bars, some energy bars, tortillas, microwave popcorn, fish sticks or other breaded frozen foods all can contain trans fat. So can some puddings and peanut butters, when used, to give a creamier consistency.

Frozen foods: Foods like pot pies, frozen pizzas and other entrees, even if labeled as lower in fat, are often made with trans fat. Very high levels can be found in packaged instant noodles like Ramen and soup cups.

Some progress is being made. In April 2004, the Kraft Foods Biscuit Division announced the introduction of three new varieties of its popular Oreo cookie will now contain zero grams of trans fat per serving. There is now a glimmer of hope in the battle to ban trans fats from all foods!

Microwave ovens have become such cooking icons of the 21st century hardly anyone ever gives them a second thought. These days very few homes or restaurants could ever imagine being without them. In fact, over 90 percent of American homes have microwave ovens. Just about everything gets popped into these handy little modern cooking devices enabling, even the most cooking - challenged person, to stave off starvation. Kids and their parents love them because they're quick and easy. The hunger for meals or snacks can be satisfied with almost instant gratification.

But is it possible millions of people are ignorantly sacrificing their health in exchange for this modern convenience? Disturbing research has shed light on the many dangers of microwave cooking. Contrary to popular belief, microwave cooking is neither natural nor healthy. In fact, it is far more dangerous to the human body than anyone could imagine. Dr. Lita Lee's book, *Health Effects of Microwave Radiation - Microwave Ovens*, states every microwave oven leaks electro-magnetic radiation, harms food and converts substances cooked in it to dangerous toxic and carcinogenic products.

It is now becoming evident they should be used as little as possible, if at all, for the following reasons.

1. Continually eating food processed from a microwave oven causes long term and permanent brain damage by "shorting out" electrical impulses in the brain [de-polarizing or de-magnetizing the brain tissue].

2. The human body cannot metabolize the unknown by-products created in microwaved food.

3. Male and female hormone production is shut down and/or altered by continually eating microwaved foods.

4. The effects of microwaved food by-products are residual within the human body.

5. Minerals, vitamins, and nutrients of all microwaved food are reduced or altered so the human body gets little or no benefit, or the human body absorbs altered compounds unable to be broken down. There is a decrease in the bioavailability of B-complex vitamins, Vitamin C, Vitamin E and essential minerals in all foods.

6. The minerals in vegetables are altered into cancerous free radicals when cooked in microwave ovens.

7. Microwaved foods cause stomach and intestinal cancerous tumors.

8. The prolonged eating of microwaved foods causes cancerous cells to increase in human blood.

9. Continual ingestion of microwaved food causes immune system deficiencies through lymph gland and blood serum alterations.

10. Eating microwaved food causes loss of memory, concentration, emotional instability, and a decrease of intelligence.

Microwave ovens are clearly not worth the risks to our children's health. They should be used only as the last resort and as infrequently as possible. Better yet, why not just give your microwave oven away?

Chapter 9
The Silent Invasion

Hormone disruptors, like silent saboteurs, have invaded the highly sensitive endocrine systems of our children. Is there any wonder why precocious puberty is a worldwide epidemic? Early puberty is a known risk for breast cancer and should be a serious concern for every mother and father. All possible precautions must be taken to safe guard our daughters and sons from unnecessary toxic exposure. No one really knows the psychological and physiological long-term consequences of early sexual development.

Think about it. Our children are accumulating chemicals in their bodies every year. For some children the effects may become evident quickly, for others it may take many years or decades.

With the red flags waving, you would think the medical profession would be in the lead warning about the sources of hormone disruptor contamination and exposure and actively encouraging parents to reduce their use of such products. After all, they are in the trenches, daily witnessing the rising number of children with precocious puberty as well as all the other health problems. They should certainly be the ones jumping up and down and yelling and screaming the loudest for something to be done.

It is, therefore, rather mind boggling a report by the Lawson Wilkins Pediatric Endocrine Society (LWPES), a nationwide network of physicians suggested that it is perfectly normal for caucasian girls as young as 7 and African American girls as young as 6 to start developing breasts! Perfectly normal? Instead of facing up to the implications of what is causing this aberration and leading the charge for causes and solutions, the medical community prefers to lower the bar or perhaps, more accurately, stick their heads in the sand. They have redefined what is considered normal to reflect current trends. How very disappointing. By claiming nothing is wrong, no fingers will be pointed and no accusations can be laid...and no feathers will be ruffled. Industries and corporations can continue to merrily go about their business of contaminating and polluting.

What Can Be Done?

Unfortunately, traditional medicine has no answers and can only address the problem by prescribing powerful, toxic drugs to totally turn off and power down the endocrine system. Presently the only thing available from traditional medical doctors is the dangerous drug, Lupron. According to the *Physician's Desk References,* Lupron has 265 possible risks and side effects, including cancer. Lupron can cause severe problems, such as tremors, seizures and memory loss. The FDA has received a wide range of reports of serious side effects, including death, suspected to be associated with the use of Lupron. However, the agency, asserts the drug's benefits outweigh the risks, and does not believe there is sufficient proof to discourage Lupron use.

From a more holistic perspective there is alot to be done. Prevention, protection and education are always the first line of action. Reduce hormone disruptors by cleaning up one's immediate living environment. Substitute as many chemical products with non-toxic ones. Eat organic food, drink filtered water and change your cooking methods.

Children with early puberty often have allergies, food intolerances, candida, digestive problems and high levels of toxins and heavy metals. These problems can undermine a child's health. It is imperative to correct these health issues because they will compromise a child's well-being putting them at greater risk of hormonal imbalances and many other serious health challenges including asthma, obesity, diabetes, compromised immunity, learning disabilities and behavioral problems.

Seek out assistance from health practitioners trained in holistic modalities. Use complimentary medical doctors, naturopathic physicians, oriental medical doctors, chiropractors, osteopaths, homeopaths and clinical nutritionists. These practitioners will be able to identify and address the underlying problems. The earlier these issues are effectively attended to, the greater the success of reversing early puberty and restoring health. Precocious puberty is a side effect of the many perils of twenty-first century living. There is much to do to insure our children do not become teens before their time.

Ways to Reduce Risk to Children

There are many things parents can do to reduce the risk of hormone disrupting influences children are exposed to.

The following are some basic guidelines.

1. Eliminate any pesticide, herbicide and insecticide use on lawns and gardens. Even some commercial compost may be contaminated with chemicals. Effective organic products are available or learn to make your own pest control formulas. Make your own organic compost.

2. Make as much of your diet organic as possible. This eliminates the toxic, hormone-disrupting chemicals sprayed on fruits and vegetables. Buy organic meat, poultry, dairy and butter free of steroid hormones and antibiotics. Organic foods have been found to contain higher amounts of vitamins and minerals.

3. Be aware. The following commercially grown fruits and vegetables contain the most pesticides: spinach strawberries, apricots,

cantaloupe, green beans, peaches, bell peppers, celery, cucumbers, cherries and grapes.

4. Glutamine rich foods help the liver remove environmental waste. They include the following foods for protection against pollution: broccoli, cauliflower and other cruciferous vegetables, asparagus, spinach, watermelon, pears, squash and potatoes.

5. Allylsulfide-containing foods like garlic, shallots, onions and chives stimulate glutathione production, a powerful antioxidant for cellular production of energy and proper immune function. Miso, a fermented soybean paste, and seaweeds remove pollution and radiation from the body.

6. Thoroughly wash non-organic fruits and vegetables with either a fruit and vegetable wash available at health food stores or soak them in an apple cider vinegar and water bath. Best selling author and clinical nutritionist, Ann Louise Gittleman highly recommends using a Clorox bath for removing bacteria, parasites, pesticides and other contaminants from food. Add a teaspoon of Clorox to one gallon of water. Soak leafy vegetables and thin-skinned fruit (berries, plums, peaches etc.) for 15 minutes; root, thick-skinned or fibrous vegetables and thick skinned fruits (oranges, bananas, apple) and poultry, fish and eggs for 20 minutes. Frozen meats (not ground meat) can be thawed in a Clorox bath for about 20

minutes for up to 5 pounds of meat. Use only Clorox since it does not contain any chlorine.

7. Use organic, toxic –free personal care products. Most deodorants, shampoos, sunscreens, skin care, body care, and baby products contain carcinogenic or toxic chemicals. Of the 2,983 chemicals used in cosmetics, at least one-third (884) of these ingredients have been reported as toxic substances.

8. Don't let children chew on soft plastic toys. Phthalates are added to soften PVC plastic toys. Plastic toys also retain pesticides that are sprayed in the house for up to two weeks. Buy unfinished wood or natural fiber toys.

9. Avoid lice and scabies shampoos containing lindane and synthetic pyrethroid. Lindane has been shown to promote tumor growth the same way estrogen did.

10. Teach your children to wash their hands frequently, not to lick their fingers or bite their nails. Since chemicals inevitably deposit on surfaces, frequent cleaning with organic cleaning products is a safe preventative measure.

11. Whenever possible, avoid buying canned foods or foods wrapped in plastic. Make sure you remove foods from packaging as soon as possible. Use glassware for oven or microwave cooking. Plastic baby bottle can also leach harmful chemicals into the formulas or drink.

12. Don't forget pet products, such as flea collars and washes, contain toxic substances which are not only dangerous to your animals but also get transferred to their owners.

13. Carefully read the labels of the foods, personal care product, household cleaners, cosmetics lawn and garden supplies and pet supplies. Become familiar with the dangerous chemicals found in such products and be willing to buy other safer brands.

14. Install a water filter. Pesticides, other chemicals, rotting leaves and other debris combine in drinking water. Heavy metals from household pipes and plumbing can be an added concern.

15. Plants are helpful for filtering chemicals from the air in your home. Even chemicals emitted from new carpets or drapes can be filtered by common household plants. For instance, Boston ferns can detoxify 1,000 micrograms of formaldehyde from the air in one hour. Other air-purifying plants include: palms, ferns, peace lilies, spider plants, ivy, dracaena and chrysanthemums

16. Exercise. Sweating eliminates all kinds of chemicals otherwise eliminated through the body's other excretory organs (the kidneys and bowel).

17. Lobby in your community to stop the spraying of hormone-disrupting chemicals in and around schools and city properties.

PART FOUR
What's Happening To Our Teenagers And Young Adults?

Chapter 1
The Pill - A Girl's Best Friend or Worst Enemy?

Life as a teenager is challenging at the best of times. Peer and social pressures, economic concerns, health problems, schoolwork, and family tensions all tilt the stress barometer into the dangerous red zone. Skipping meals, eating junk food and starvation dieting are a way of life for teenagers. More than ever, teenagers seem to be burning the candle at both ends.

The behaviors and decisions teenagers make directly affect their physical and emotional health. As a result, teenage girls' hormonal health is under siege. Premenstrual Syndrome (PMS), painful periods, irregular or absent periods, ovarian cysts, polycystic ovaries, fibrocystic breast disease (lumpy, painful breasts) endometriosis, hormonal migraines, allergies, fatigue and mood swings are occurring in young women at epidemic rates. Many girls try to ignore their health problems hoping they will disappear. Others schedule an appointment with their doctors. Odds are they will leave the office with either a prescription for a hormonal contraceptive or other medication.

What women are rarely told and, usually fail to understand, is hormonal imbalances, in whatever way the symptoms may be manifesting, are really powerful red flags warning them their health is being seriously compromised and undermined. Reliance on drugs to manage symptoms or regulate functions can be a recipe for disaster.

There is no doubt doctors consider the pill the most popular solution to address a long list of teenagers' hormonal difficulties. There are a plethora of options: the combined low dose pill made with estrogen and progestin, the patch, the progestin mini pill, and the three year implant or injection. Far beyond it's initial purpose as a contraceptive drug for short term use, the pill has become the darling of the medical world for treating just about any female hormonal problem.

To date, the pill is prescribed to help teenagers attack acne, to regulate their periods, to eliminate painful periods, to regain missing periods, to treat PMS, endometriosis, heavy bleeding, ovarian cysts and polycystic ovaries. There is even a popular trend promoted by doctors encouraging young women to eliminate menstruation by using a new continuous low dose pill. As the drug companies create marketing campaigns extolling the pill's ever growing virtues and benefits directly to doctors, as well as young women, should we be cheering for this 21st century 'miracle' or loudly ringing the alarm bells?

The Birth of the Birth Control Pill

A revolution was about to begin when the birth control pill arrived on the scene in 1960. It heralded an era that would emancipate fertile women from the burden of unwanted pregnancies and open the door to greater equality and freedom. For more than 40 years about 200 million women around the world have chosen the pill as their preferred method of contraception. This 'medical miracle' has enlisted almost 90 percent of Western women of reproductive age on some kind of contraceptive at some time in their lives.

The pill has been proclaimed as one of the most studied drugs in history. In its early days, it was said the pill was safer than pregnancy. After four decades of experimentation (unfortunately on the unsuspecting pill users), we are told safe dosages are, at last, finally known. However, as the thin veneer of advertising hype, pharmaceutical cover-ups and sanitized clinical trials is peeled away, another picture emerges revealing the devastating consequences to women's health and well-being from the use of steroid hormones found in the pill.

Far from safe and risk-free, it is now recognized these steroid hormones are, in reality, dangerous and potentially life-threatening steroid drugs causing grave harm to women. Most women taking the contraceptive pill have very little knowledge about what they are putting into their bodies or its dangerous potential side-effects. A soaring incidence of breast and cervical cancers, strokes, cardiovascular disease, blood clots, impaired immunity, infertility osteoporosis, and major nutritional imbalances are only some of the conditions undeniably linked to these hormones.

The Pill's Hidden Agenda

In the 1950's, the specter of a world doomed by overpopulation was alarming scientists and governments in the industrialized West. Their fear began a frantic rush to control populations. This coincided with the discovery of a relatively inexpensive process for making synthetic estrogens and synthetic progesterone, known as progestins. These are the main ingredients of contraceptives known as the combined pill.

As early as 1932, animal experiments revealed estrogen and progestins could cause cancer of the breast, uterus, ovaries and pituitary glands. The pill, however, was believed to be an effective solution to the looming world crisis.

In spite of the discovered dangers, the decision was taken to go ahead with clinical trials of the pill. Since it was then common knowledge estrogens could cause breast cancer, the original pill trials in America used a single ingredient, progestins. When 'pure' progestins were given, women complained of too much bleeding. It was then realized a regular monthly period required the addition of estrogen. Dr. John Rock and Dr. Gregory Pincus tried out the first 'Pincus Pill' in the 1950s on a Harvard volunteer group and on some chronically ill mental patients. Both men and women took a high dose form of Envoid (10mg), which was more than enough to stop ovulation in women and sperm production in men.

When some of the men in the study displayed shrunken testicles, all further trials with the 'male pill' were unceremoniously abandoned. The researchers unanimously agreed any 'male pill' would have to be proven safe before experiments could proceed. No such caveat about the 'female pill' was ever given to safeguard the health of women.

Nobel Laureate Frederick Robbins expressed the prevailing attitude of the time stating, "the dangers of the over-population are so great, we may have to use certain techniques of conception control may entail considerable risk to the individual woman".

And considerable risks they did contain. Envoid, the first oral contraceptive, was given a clean bill of health by the FDA in 1960 on the basis of one clinical study which involved only 132 Puerto Rican women who had taken the pill for a year or longer. Five died during the study, yet no effort was made to determine the cause of their deaths. Not surprisingly, the initial trials were flawed and inadequate. In spite of what should have been a serious warning, the pill was promoted with all the enthusiasm the pharmaceutical companies could muster,

Although it was known early on the pill caused blood clots, it wasn't until the mid-1970s that the death toll for young women from heart attacks and strokes began to get public attention. Pill users were 11 times more likely to have thrombo-embolisms. Prophetic warnings from some doctors regarding the widespread use of oral contraceptives would give rise to health hazards on a scale previously unknown in medicine were coming true.

It is evident the early reassurances by the government and pharmaceutical companies were lies. A study by the U.S. Department of Health and Human Services disclosed more than 70 percent of oral contraceptive advertising to doctors are 'misleading or unbalanced' - making contraceptives the most 'deceptively advertised' category of prescription drug.[1]

While many variations of the pill have successfully been accepted into the lifestyle of millions of women, the fact remains the long term effects from artificially altering a woman's hormonal and reproductive life bodes ill for the health of women. Dr. David Clark, neurologist for the University of Kentucky School of Medicine expressed the real situation when he said, "The pill allows experiments on the general population that would never be allowed as a planned experiment."[2] How generous of women to be donating their bodies to medical science even if no informed consent was ever given!

By 1975 the devastating effects of young women dying from blood clots and heart attacks caused public outrage. The ensuing pressure from consumer groups convinced the FDA Commissioner to propose oral contraceptives be accompanied by package inserts. He suggested providing full length comprehensive warnings about possible side-effects of the recommended dosage. It was expected there would be opposition from manufacturers. What was not anticipated, however, were the heated attacks from the American Medical Association and the American College of Obstetrician and Gynecologists. It seemed since the medical profession did not want to inform women of the risks, no one else should either.

Believing the pill is perfectly safe and harmless, women are lulled into a false sense of security. Unfortunately, nothing could be further from the truth.

Hormones are very powerful substances. Begin tampering with nature's finely tuned messengers of life's processes and you are asking for trouble. This is especially true for young women.

Hormones not only direct and determine physiological processes but influence emotional and psychological states. Besides controlling sexual development, function, and fertility, hormones also help to control growth and muscle building, regulate the digestive system, blood sugar levels, blood pressure and fluid balance.

Hormones also hold the key to subjective feelings and changes in blood chemistry associated with stress. Hormonal imbalances not only create a myriad of health problems and diseases, but can also undermine self-esteem, a sense of well-being, emotional balance and mental acuity.

Two of the most significant reproductive hormones in a woman's body are estrogen and progesterone. Nature has choreographed these two hormones to work together with exquisite timing and balance. Estrogen, produced in the first half of a cycle, is responsible for the sexual development of females, the growth of breasts, the development of the reproductive system and the shape of the female body. It also stimulates the growth of cells preparing the endometrial lining for fertilization each month. The target organs of the breast, uterus, ovaries and the skin are particularly sensitive to estrogen.

Progesterone, on the other hand, halts estrogen's effect of rapid cell growth. It also develops the proliferative lining of the uterus ensuring the implantation of a fertilized egg (it is the pro-gestation hormone). Progesterone is known as a precursor hormone since estrogen (made up of estradiol, estrone and estriol), testosterone and the stress hormones are all synthesized from it. Progesterone is not only a sex hormone but is also intricately involved in maintaining many of the body's other vital physiological functions.

Hormones made by the body are called endogenous, while those from outside sources such as found in foods, chemicals or in prescription drugs are called exogenous. Most estrogens, whether natural or synthetic like those found in the pill, still act exactly like estrogens. All exogenous hormones tend to cause biochemical stress in the body.[1]

When a woman is pregnant, levels of estrogen and progesterone rise and further egg production is stopped. The hormones levels continue to rise during pregnancy signaling the pituitary gland secreting egg stimulating hormones. The hormones in the pill actually mimic this effect and continually fool the brain into thinking that pregnancy has occurred. Thus, ovulation is suppressed.

The present day oral contraceptives are made up of varying doses of estrogen-progestin formulations (the combination pill, or patch) or progestin only products (the mini pill, injections and implants such as Depo-Provera and Implanon.)

So, how does really work? It literally stops natural menstruation. Bleeding only occurs each month because the synthetic hormones are not taken for the last seven days of the cycle causing the uterine lining to shed. The bleeding occuring at this time is more accurately termed 'withdrawal bleeding' not menstruation. In fact, there is nothing natural about taking the pill. The action of the pill is actually the female form of 'castration' because it stops the natural reproductive cycle, turning off the ovaries. There is also the risk a woman's ovaries may become permanently damaged resulting in infertility.

Fabio Bertarelli, a Swiss billionaire who manufacturers 70 percent of the world's fertility drugs has admitted. "Our usual customers are women over 30 who have been taking birth-control pills since they were teenagers or in their early 20's." In 1995, 6.2 million women in the U.S. had fertility problems, compared to 4.5 million in 1982 and this number could be as high as 7.7 million women in 2025".[2] Business is certainly booming for the fertility business.

Both the progestin-only and estrogen-progesterone formulations act to cause alterations to the lining of the womb. They convert the proliferative nature of the endometrium, which is naturally designed to accept and sustain a fertilized ovum, to a secretory endometrium which is a thin, devasculating lining, physiologically unreceptive to receiving and sustaining a fetus. The pill also causes changes to the movement of the fallopian tubes. It alters the time taken for the passage of the ovum down the fallopian tube, reducing the possibility of an egg being fertilized. It also contributes to the high incidence of ectopic (the fertilized egg remains in the fallopian tube) pregnancies.

Clearly, when you interfer with a woman's hormones you are tampering with her most sensitive physiological and psychological processes. By interfering with these vital processes, many profound changes are initiated in a woman's body. Some are long term and can ultimately result is serious health problems.

Minor Side Effects

Allergic reactions
Breakthrough bleeding
Decreased immune system function
Disturbances in liver function
Eye disorders
Swelling of optic nerve, contact lens intolerance and corneal inflammation
Facial and body hair growth
Fluid retention and bloating
Fungal infections and tinea
Hair loss
Hayfever, asthma, skin rashes
Loss of libido

Lumpy or tender breasts
Migraines
Nausea
Psychological and emotional disorders,
Depression, mood changes
Secretions from the breast
Skin discoloration
Suicide is much more common among pill-users
than those using other forms of contraception
Weight gain
Systemic candida infection
Urinary tract infection
Venereal warts
Vaginal discharges
Varicose veins

Major Side Effects

Disturbance to blood-sugar metabolism
Increased risk of stroke
Increased risk of artery hardening
Increased risk of blood clots
Increased risk of gall bladder disease
Liver tumors
Risk of cancer of the endometrium, cervix, ovaries,
breast, liver, skin and lungs
Significant risk of ectopic pregnancy
Strong risk of rapid development of pre-existing
cancers and progression to cancer of abnormal cells
Three-to-six fold increase in risk of heart attacks
Osteoporosis

Early prophetic warnings were issued about the dangers of the pill. In 1961 Sir Charles Dodd, president of the Royal College of Physicians announced, "Women who have continuous treatment with the contraceptive pill have an entirely different hormonal background due to pituitary inhibition. One cannot help but wonder what will happen if this state of affairs is allowed to continue."[1]

Sir Charles should know since he and his colleagues discovered the first non-steroid estrogen compound known as diethylstilbestrol (DES). Although a synthetic compound, it locked into the estrogen receptors so exactly, the cell was fooled into thinking the bodies own estrogens were stimulating activity. Sir Charles gave stern warnings of stilboestrol's power and cautioned against its unrestricted use.

Synthetic progesterone, known as progestin, was first made in 1944 by a long and complicated method. Progestins are between 500 and 1,000 times more powerful than the progesterone made using the body.

For the best part of two centuries it has been known sex hormones cause cancer in hormone-dependent tissues. In 1940, pharmaceutical estrogenic chemicals were first appearing on the market, and American women's lifetime risk of breast cancer was 1 in 20. Presently, women's lifetime risk is now 1 in 7.

"Every study shows an increase now", confirms Carol Ann Rinzler, author of *Estrogens and Breast Cancer*. She is especially worried about the youngest users who may take the pill for four years or longer prior to birth of their first child. These young women, she explains, are at the highest risk of cancer from the pill and the highest risk of sexually transmitted diseases. Teenagers are particularly vulnerable to the potent artificial steroid drugs contained in the pill, which can cause 150 different chemical changes in a girl's body.

By the mid 1970's, a new test allowing doctors to identify

estrogen-dependent tumors. This test determined approximately 70 percent of breast cancers contained cell chains hooked up with estrogen molecules. Such tumors, called estrogen receptor positive or ER+, grow when exposed to estrogen and shrink when their source of estrogen is withdrawn.

This new technology has allowed epidemiological researchers to examine which kinds of breast cancer tumors are increasing. In 1990, a study based on information from the Kaiser Permanente tumor registry in the U.S., revealed from 1974 to 1985, the incidence of ER+ breast tumors nationwide rose 131 per cent.[2] Clearly, the influence of estrogen fuels breast cancer. So do progestins. Some of the synthetic progestins have estrogenic activity, causing persistent stimulation to breast tissue.

Dr. Max Cutler, a highly respected Los Angeles surgeon gave a chilling testimony at a U.S. Senate Hearing investigating the pill. This foremost authority on breast cancer had been performing microscopic studies of biopsy material from patients who had taken oral contraceptives. "I have a series of patients who have had two or three breast biopsies. In some, the biopsies were performed before the patient started to take the contraceptive pill. A second or third biopsy was performed after the patient had been on the pill for several years. Studying surgical specimens under these circumstances presents a unique opportunity to observe the tissue changes."[3]

As Dr. Cutler feared, his biopsies revealed "increased cellular activity, reflecting the stimulating effects of the estrogen." He testified "the risk is a potential time bomb with a fuse at least 15 to 20 years in length. This gamble is difficult to justify because of the large numbers of women at risk. The available evidence indicates a relationship between the steroid hormones and the induction of breast cancer, and suggests that this relationship is dose and time-related. The higher the dose given and the longer the exposure, the greater the number of cancers were produced in animals."[4]

By the late 1980's studies began to reveal the full extent of the pill/breast cancer link. A major study in the *Lancet* in 1989 found "there was a highly significant trend in risk of breast cancer with the total duration of oral contraceptives."[5] Women using the pill for 49-96 months had a 43 percent greater risk of breast cancer and users for more than 97 months had a 74 percent greater risk.

This research was further backed up by a paper published in the *American Journal of Epidemiology* which reported women who were on the pill for at least 4 to 10 years beginning early in life have a 40-70 percent greater risk of premenopausal breast cancer than do women who were never on the pill.[6]

Since the breast tissue of young girls is still developing, it is particularly sensitive to the over-stimulation from estrogen. The younger a girl is, the more stem cells (undeveloped cells vulnerable to damage by cancer-causing agents) she has in her breast tissue. Studies have found women who took the pill before the age of 20 and were later diagnosed with breast cancer have tumors with the worse prognoses than do breast cancer patients who started taking the pill at a later age or had not previously taken it. Even more alarming, the younger the women were at the time of diagnosis, the greater the possibility they would be dead within five years. It was also shown the pill caused chromosomal aberrations in breast tissue. They not only potentially damage DNA but also reduce the body's capacity to protect and repair it.[7]

In 1977 norethisterone, the most common progestin in progestin–estrogen combination oral contraceptives, and other synthetic progestins used for injections and implants, was listed as known human carcinogens.[8]

Studies continued and the debates raged until December 2002 when the US government published its *Report on Carcinogens*. The report stated all steroidal estrogens found in hormone replacement therapy and oral contraceptives are "known human carcinogens", contributing to hormone dependent cancers, in particular, breast cancer, uterine cancer and ovarian cancer.[9]

The gravity of this finding cannot be overstated: all estrogens have now been proven, unequivocally, to fuel cancer! The other popular progestin, medroxyprogesterone acetate, better known as Provera (used in HRT) or the contraceptive injection, Depo-Provera, also has its place in the *Fourth Report on Carcinogens*. Depo-Provera should be of great concern to women. The *British Medical Journal* (1989) reported women who used it before the age of 25 increased their relative risk of breast cancer by 50 percent and for women using it for six or more years; their risk was raised significantly to 320 percent.[10]

There is now overwhelming evidence when teenage girls take birth control pills or progestin-only forms of birth control, they increase their risk of breast cancer. The decision to use any form of birth control, especially when prescribed for hormonal imbalance, should be reconsidered. When girls between the ages of 13-21 use birth control pills, their risk of breast cancer increases by as much as 600 percent.[11]

The prevailing myth that the pill is a safe and natural way to correct hormonal imbalances has lead to its widespread use in correcting teenager's menstrual cycles or alleviating painful periods. Puberty has now been medicalized. Even though nature often requires several years to balance out a teenager's menstrual cycle, girls, as young as 13, complaining of menstrual irregularities or even acne are readily prescribed the pill.

Little do these teenagers or their parents realize they are traveling down a road putting them at risk of aggressive pre-menopausal breast cancer.

The pill has a powerful effect on the way the body utilizes important nutrients. In some cases it significantly reduces important vitamin and mineral levels and in other cases it raises their levels. Altering the availability and use of these vital nutrients results in major imbalances in the body with potentially serious and long-term consequences.

One of the most important minerals for the body is zinc. Zinc is crucial for the growth and division of cells, for brain development and function and for the normal functioning of every single cell.

Unfortunately, zinc levels are radically affected by hormones. According to researcher Dr. Ellen Grant, "Zinc deficiency affects nearly all my patients who have taken hormones, sometimes even including those who are already taking supplements if their absorption is also impaired."[1]

Zinc-deficiency causes ovulation and sex hormone production to be impaired and affects sexual desire and fertility. Taking extra hormones can increase these faults. Both cell and blood zinc levels are lowered by estrogen and progestins. The pill also tends to increase copper levels. It is acknowledged that low zinc and high copper causes mental turmoil, mood swings, irritability and in extreme cases schizophrenia.

Zinc is essential for fetal brain development. Vitamin and mineral deficiencies can occur in women, not only while they are taking the pill, but for a long time after. This means even though a woman has been off the pill for some time, the deficiencies can remain. In the case of zinc, without adequate levels, the healthy development of a growing fetus can be compromised. Healthy zinc levels are especially important in early pregnancy to prevent congenital deformities.

Other pill-induced deficiencies can cause serious birth deformities. For instance, folic acid deficiencies have been linked to limb defects and Down Syndrome. Folic acid is essential for protecting DNA from damage. There is a much higher incidence of stillbirths, miscarriages and birth defects, such as heart abnormalities, occurring in women who have conceived within a month of coming off the pill.[2] While the mini-pill, or progestin-only pill, does not suppress ovulation, it causes changes in the lining of the womb and cervical mucus, which also interferes with the passage of the egg into the fallopian tubes leading to an increased risk of ectopic pregnancies. It is also prescribed for lactating mothers and has been shown to severely deplete nutrients in the milk and causes progestins to find their way into mother's milk. These hormones are known to act on the hypothalamus and may masculinize a female infant and contribute to neo-natal jaundice.

Vitamin and Mineral Imbalances Caused by the Pill

The following is a list of vitamin and mineral imbalances caused by the pill:[3]

> *Vitamin A* (**Retinol**) - Levels in the blood are increased when on the pill. Whether this means the body's turnover of this vitamin is higher (requiring a higher level of ingestion) as there is less stored in the liver, or whether there is a greater availability to the tissues is not yet clear. Vitamin A is needed for the healthy functioning of the eyes. Increased susceptibility to infections, dry and scaly skin, lack of appetite and vigor, defective teeth and gums and retarded growth are also reported with Vitamin A deficiencies. Vitamin A is also an important anti-oxidant and anti-cancer vitamin, and best taken as beta-carotene, to avoid toxicity.

Vitamin B (Thiamine) - There is a probability pill takers are deficient in this vitamin. Side-effects include fatigue, weakness, insomnia, vague aches and pains, weight loss, depression, irritability, lack of initiative, constipation, over sensitivity to noise, loss of appetite and circulatory problems.

Vitamin B2 (Riboflavin) - Requirements of the body are raised by use of the pill, leading to deficiencies. Side effects include gum and mouth infections, dizziness, depression, eye irritation, skin problems and dandruff.

Vitamin B6 (Pyridoxine) - Depletion varies from marginal to severe. Side effects include nausea, low stress tolerance, lethargy, anxiety, depression, weakness, nervousness, emotional flare-ups, fatigue, insomnia, mild paranoia, skin eruptions, loss of muscular control, eye problems, herpes infection and edema (fluid retention). Vitamin B6 is needed to help convert tryptophan to serotonin (a brain compound that affects moods, sleep patterns, psychological drive and sexual desire), to normalize sugar metabolism and to help prevent blood clots forming.

Folic Acid - Levels are reduced on the pill. Folic acid is required by the body to facilitate cell division. Low levels cause a much higher risk of birth defects, including neural tube defects, spina bifida, deformed limbs and Downs Syndome. Deficiencies can also lead to anemia.

Vitamin B12 (**Cobalamine**) - Levels in the blood are lowered in pill users, especially vegetarians. Resulting in anemia, sore tongue, weight loss and depression.

Vitamin C (**Ascorbic acid**) - Levels are reduced on the pill by up to 30 per cent, worsened by smoking, stress, high pollution levels, infections and some medications. The effectiveness of vitamin C supplementation can also be reduced. This can result in bruising, bleeding gums, eye problems, loss of appetite, muscular weakness, anaemia, fatigue and lowered immune response. This vitamin is also necessary for the production of sex hormones, something your body will have to start doing for itself when you come off the pill. A deficiency can make it even harder for your body to resume normal production.

Vitamin E (**Alpha Tocopherol**) - The need for vitamin E is increased while taking the pill (this vitamin helps to normalize estrogen levels). Effects include anaemia, muscle degeneration, subsequent low fertility, changes in the menstrual cycle, and hot flushes. It helps offset the possible carcinogenic effect of the estrogen, as does selenium, which plays a part in vitamin E absorption and is decreased by the pill.

Vitamin K (**Menadione**) - Higher levels may lead to blood clot formations.

Taurine - Reduces levels of the amino acid necessary for good memory.

Tyrosine - Reduces levels of the amino acid necessary for the healthy functioning of the thyroid gland.

Copper - Absorption is increased raising the need for vitamin C, disrupting the zinc/copper balance and leading to insomnia, depression, migraine, hair loss, high blood pressure and blood clots.

Magnesium - Lowers levels, which can result in kidney stones, muscle cramps, nervous irritability, confusion, depression, impaired protein metabolism and premature wrinkles.

Selenium - Lowers levels of this powerful antioxidant mineral. Slows down aging and provides protection against cancer and mercury toxicity.

Zinc - Levels are significantly lowered. This can lead to diabetes, poor resistance to infection, skin infections, and reduced fertility. This mineral is crucial for normal growth, cell division, tissue repair, and during pregnancy, in over 200 enzyme systems in the body, and is crucial for the development of brain function and a competent immune system. Long-term pill users can find it difficult to build back their zinc status to an adequate level.

Prostaglandins - Levels of certain prostaglandins are lower on the pill. These are normally made from essential fatty acids; using zinc as a catalyst, and decrease tendencies to clot formations.

Blood Lipids - Low density lipids, cholesterol and triglycerides are increased on the pill.

Serum Proteins - Are altered by the pill.

It is most important to stop taking the pill and replenish nutrients at least three to six months before attempting to conceive.

Necessary Nutrients

Oral contraceptives create certain nutrient deficiencies and it is of utmost importance to supplement with appropriate vitamins, minerals and other essential nutrients.

Most of the B vitamins, particularly pyridoxine (B6) and folic acid, are needed in higher amounts when birth control pills are taken. Copper levels usually rise, and zinc levels often fall. Thus, more zinc is needed as well. An increased need for vitamins C, E, and K may also result from the use of birth control pills.

Birth control pills cause imbalance in the ph of the vagina leading to increased susceptibility to infection. Extra ascorbic acid, 1-2 grams per day, may help balance the acid environment and prevent this problem. The increased blood levels of copper generated by oral contraceptive use may contribute to depression and emotional symptoms; additional manganese and zinc may reverse these symptoms.

Depression caused by the pill is a neuro-chemical reaction to hormones and from a lack of a women's own superior hormones i.e. estradiol and natural progesterone. Iron levels may also rise, and less iron may be required because the pill often reduces the amount of menstrual blood loss.

Since the liver metabolizes oral contraceptives before being eliminated, a diet low in other liver irritants such as alcohol, caffeine, pesticides and preservative chemicals in foods should be followed. Cutting down on refined foods and sugary treats is also suggested. These foods are "empty" calories and may cause further nutrient depletion. Avoiding nicotine and fried foods is also a good idea to prevent further vascular irritation. Teenage girls on the pill must also be particularly careful to avoid nutritional deficiencies. Women would be well advised to take supportive nutritional supplements. Adequate intake of the antioxidant nutrients, such as vitamins C and E, selenium, and beta-carotene, can help reduce potential toxicity of oral contraceptives. The herb, milk thistle, may be especially helpful.

A high-nutrient diet is the best prevention for problems. High quality protein sources and nutritious foods (whole grains, vegetables, nuts, and seeds) are important. Eating lots of vegetables is the best way to prevent many mineral deficits and also maintain weight. Several teaspoons of cold-pressed oil, particularly olive oil and flax seed oil, should also be used daily to ensure the intake of the essential fatty acids. The above-mentioned foods, along with protein intake from eggs, fish, poultry, raw dairy foods, and legumes, are a sensible approach. Whenever possible, foods should be organically grown.

If oral contraceptives are being used, it is recommended the intake of the following nutrients be added or increased to the levels listed:

Nutrient	Daily Amounts (in 1 or 2 doses)
Vitamin B6	50-100 mg
Vitamin B12	50-200 mcg
Folic acid	60-800 mcg
Vitamin E	400-600 IUs
Vitamin C	1-3 g
Zinc	20-40 mg
Essential Fatty Acids found in olive or flax seed	
Oils	1-2 teaspoons
Calcium	600-1,000 mg
Chromium	200-400 mcg
Copper	1-2 mg
Iron	15-20 mg
Magnesium	400- 600 mg
Manganese	5-10 mg
Selenium	150-300 mcg
Zinc	30-60mg

Other B vitamins can also be increased and additional 25mg to balance out the B complex. More antioxidants also help reduce the deleterious effects of the drugs. These include beta-carotene, selenium, and the amino acid L-cysteine.

Copper intake in supplements should be limited to 1 mg., though the increased zinc intake will help lower copper levels. Whole grains, nuts, seeds, and vegetables will ensure copper requirements are met. Iron supplements may be decreased somewhat with use of birth control pills unless the menstrual periods are heavy or there is anemia.

The Pill and Infertility

Infertility is a cause of growing concern around the world.

There are presently 6.4 million infertile American women. There is no doubt the pill is a major contributing factor to declining fertility.

In *The Couples Guide to Infertility*, Dr. Gary S. Berger has found, "Long-term pill users may not menstruate or ovulate after they stop using the pill. This condition, known as post-pill amenorrhea, occurs because the pill disrupts the natural rhythmic flow of hormones from the hypothalamus to the pituitary to the ovaries."

What is even more alarming is the return to ovulation when the pill is stopped does not mean a woman has returned to fertility. The pill can damage the glands producing the cervical mucus necessary for fertilization. There may also be an over stimulation of the specific cervical mucus which impedes sperm motility. These two interlinked actions of the pill on mucus production can cause serious delay, if not cessation, of fertility.

In the majority of women, impairment of fertility usually diminishes with time. Post-pill fertility may be abetted by natural medicines to help detoxify the body and stimulate normal functioning.

The Pill and Sexually Transmitted Diseases

Sexually transmitted diseases have grown so prevalent the U.S. Center for Disease Control issued a startling new recommendation in 1991: "Use barrier methods. Use condoms, diaphragms and/or vaginal spermicides even if contraception is not needed."[4] It was not only the fear of AIDS prompting this advisory but the galloping increase in infections such as chlamydia, which can create pelvic inflammatory disease and infertility. The CDC estimates one million American women experience Pelvic Inflammatory Disease (PID) each year; 50

per cent become sterile after three episodes, 12 per cent after just one.

The sexual freedom the pill initiated was also responsible for the present epidemic of STD's. On the one hand, the pill increases the stickiness of cervical mucus, and slows the ascent of diseases into the uterus, fallopian tubes and ovaries. On the other hand, the pill increases the risk of infectious conditions such as chlamydia. Chlamydia is a microscopic organism; not bacteria, viruses or fungi. It causes non-gonococcal urethritis, a chlamydia infection passed on through intercourse, with symptoms of painful urinations and a watery discharge leading to PID and infertility.

The great cycles and rhythms of nature are among the most fundamental realities of physical life. A woman's body and psyche are intimately woven into these eternal cycles of Life. We are just beginning to realize the price we have paid for being part of a culture where fast food, fast cures and fast sex predominate. Certainly the long-term effects of the pill is still to be fully determined. Is it worth the price women must pay in terms of their physical, emotional and mental health for the over use of this form of contraception, as a therapeutic treatment?

Other Birth Control Choices

The use of the pill for birth control has been around for more than four generations. Women have come to rely upon it, assuming it is effective and safe. Such is not the case. Many women believe the choice is either the pill or pregnancy. Fortunately, there are other alternatives

Most women will ask, "Well, just what are the natural alternatives to the pill?" The answer to that question requires a woman to make a deeper commitment to the understanding of the workings of her body and her natural cycles. It's learning about the various indications of fertile and non-fertile times. Owning one's fertility means to have an intimate relationship with one's own body. It requires taking responsibility for sexual intercourse, to have a sense of ones self-worth, and requires the ability to communicate with an understanding and receptive partner. It is certainly a totally different approach from the way most women address the issues of contraception sexual relationships. As women move into a greater acceptance and expression of their innate power, so too must they regain authority over their reproductive cycles.

If a woman's choice is to continue using the pill, it is recommended to take a break from the pill after several years in order to insure natural fertility cycles. It is also advised to seek consultation with qualified complimentary practitioners who can assess, not only nutritional needs, but correct imbalances. The pill can interfere with the healthy functioning of the liver, pancreas, thyroid, digestive system, ovaries, immunity and vascular systems.

There are many natural birth control tools that offer a woman effective and safe contraceptive freedom. Natural fertility awareness programs are options. Methods are based on a woman's daily observance and charting her fertility signals (the waking temperature, cervical fluids, and cervix changes). Once she learns to read her fertility charts, a woman can tell whether or not she's ovulating, when she's fertile, if she's pregnant, if she's prone to miscarriage or ovarian cysts, and more. During her fertile times, she can choose from a variety of barrier methods, such as the condom, diaphragm, cervical cap or a spermicidal sponge.

There are also natural fertility tools, which incorporate various methods to naturally monitor fertile and non-fertile times rather than overriding or manipulating them. One of the best of these fertility testers is called an Ovu-tech, a device the size of a lipstick tube having a small microscopic lens at one end and a light at the other. If you are just about to become fertile, or if you are fertile, you will easily see a beautiful crystalline ferning pattern under the microscope when applying saliva to the lens. This is an easy and convenient way to monitor hormonal changes and enhance awareness of your menstrual cycle. If you track your cycles and fertility on a calendar, there will be a keen awareness of where you are in your monthly cycle. Whether you are trying to conceive, avoid conception, or charting your cycles, the Ovu-Tech is an inexpensive and reusable tool for fertility awareness. The Ovu-Tech should always be used in conjunction with charting temperature, cervical changes and mucus secretions.

The sentiment menstruation is a disease—or at least an unwelcomed and unsafe physiological process—seems to reflect a growing trend among the pharmacuetical and medical professions. They promote new scientific developments that can supposedly liberate women from their age-long debilitation. Leading the charge to stamp out menstruation is the work of Dr Elsimar Coutinho, Professor of Gynecology, Obstetrics and Human Reproduction in Brazil, as recounted in his book, *Is Menstruation Obsolete?* Dr Coutinho argues regular monthly bleeding is not the "natural" state of women and it actually places them at risk of several medical conditions of varying severity. The author maintains while menstruation may be culturally significant, it is not medically meaningful. He asserts prehistoric women had fewer than 160 periods in their lifetime. (The mind boggles at how rigorous the scientific method arrived as such conclusions!) On the other hand, modern women, who start menstruating earlier and spend less time pregnant, have more than 400 menstrual cycles.

As a self-proclaimed champion of women's freedom, Dr. Coutinho believes 21st century women should be able to choose the timing and frequency of their periods, just as they can now choose the timing and frequency of pregnancy. From a medical point of view he sees menstruation as a failed process, having no beneficial effects. He believes it can be harmful to women's health.

In a nutshell, Dr Coutinho's work suggests the most medically advanced "treatment" for menstruation should be its total cessation in all women of reproductive age. He is the spearhead of a popular trend to eliminate menstrual cycles.

The intricate and profoundly complicated female reproductive system, which has undergone many thousands of years of evolutionary fine-tuning, has now been declared obsolete. Like a top-class magician, medical science now professes the rationale and means to make menstruation disappear completely.

The solution is simple: give all women a continuous low-dose birth control pill!

Dr Coutinho's theory has many physicians and researchers agreeing there's no reason why women can't opt for fewer periods by extending the use of the pill. Whether for easing health problems eliminating the inconvenience and messiness or reduce the expense of menstruation, the pill can now be taken continuously for 84 days followed by a seven-day break. Using this method, women will only have a bleed four times a year!

The new continuous contraceptive pill Seasonale, which has recently made its debut, is the pharmaceutical's answer to menstrual obsolescence.

Needless to say, the pathologizing of women's menstrual cycles and hormonal imbalances through the pervasive and persuasive advertising campaigns, initiated by both the medical profession and pharmaceutical industries, is seriously jeopardizing the physical and emotional well-being of young women.

With the arrival of the continuous low dose pill, normal menstrual cycles are now fair game for drug treatment. This has great appeal to young women, who have been brainwashed into believing that menstrual cycles are indeed a painful curse, and a great inconvenience.

Nutritionally depleted diets, stress and environmental toxins (the real culprits of menstrual irregularities and hormonal imbalances) have been all but ignored by doctors. Why not just use a quick fix to shut the whole system down? Take a pill! Haven't we been here before?

Reminiscent of recent HRT revelations, the mass prescribing of the continuous low dose pill, without any long-term studies undertaken, amounts to a dangerous experiment being conducted on young women.

Unfortunately, it's not only the obsolescence of menstrual cycles the drug companies have on their agenda. There is another way young women are being pathologized and medicalized for their natural cycles, which can put them in jeopardy of breast cancer and other serious problems.

The pharmaceutical giant Eli Lilly is promoting its new drug, Sarafem, as a miracle pill for women suffering with a new "mental disorder" called premenstrual dysphoric disorder (PMDD). Never heard of it? It's no surprise, since it was only concocted as a psychiatric disorder a few years ago.

PMDD, purported to affect 3–10 percent of all menstruating women, is actually the new and improved version of premenstrual syndrome (PMS). To be diagnosed with PMDD, a woman must experience five or more of the following PMDD symptoms: depressed mood, anxiety, decreased interest in activities, feeling sad, hopeless, self-deprecating, tense, anxious or "on edge", persistent irritability, anger, increased interpersonal conflicts, fatigue, lethargic or lacking in energy, marked changes in appetite, a subjective feeling of being overwhelmed or out of control, and physical symptoms such as breast tenderness, swelling or bloating.

What teenage girl (or their mothers, for that matter) couldn't relate to at least five of the so-called PMDD symptoms?

The pharmaceutical giant Eli Lilly has come to the rescue. It reports, "Doctors can treat PMDD with a pretty pink-and-lavender pill called Sarafem—the first prescription medication for PMDD".

Actually, Sarafem is better known by another name, Prozac!

It is no coincidence the year Sarafem was listed as the only approved drug for this new female 'mental disorder', coincided was the year the patent on Prozac ran out. However, with the acceptance of the Prozac clone, Sarafem Lilly's patent on Prozac was extended another seven years.

Not to be left out in the cold, the makers of Zoloft, Celexa and Paxil, similar antidepressants known as serotonin reuptake inhibitors, or SSRIs, have followed suit.

Are women, once again, being manipulated, misinformed and mistreated in order to fill the drug companies' coffers?

A Strong Warning About Antidepressants

There is an even more draconian side to this. Researchers in Canada, found women who took Paxil saw their risk of breast cancer increase sevenfold![1] That's 700 percent!

Further studies have shown Prozac not only promotes tumors but causes proliferation of malignant cells by blocking the body's innate ability to kill tumor cells. There is mounting evidence these drugs can cause breast cancer and other forms of cancer such as brain cancer.[2] SSRIs are also endocrine disrupters and increased estrogen levels, further exacerbates estrogen excess conditions such as PMS, ovarian cysts, endometriosis, and polycystic ovaries.

Other side effects include: neurological disorders such as disfiguring facial and whole-body tics and sexual dysfunction. Debilitating withdrawal symptoms include visual hallucinations, electric shock–like sensations in the brain, dizziness, nausea and anxiety. The SSRIs possess another trait: they have the ability to turn normal people into raging suicidal murderers.

Three years before Prozac was approved, the FDA had such serious reservations about Prozac's safety, the antidepressants approval was refused. Studies showed previously non-suicidal patients who took the drug had a fivefold higher rate of suicide and suicide attempts than those on older anti-depressants. The British government has recently banned Paxil for adolescents because of scientific studies linking it to increased suicides rates. The FDA has issued a health warning for 10 anti-depressant drugs and their suicide links but still allows them to be prescribed to children and adolescents.

In addition to diagnosing young women with PMDD, the growing incidence of depression and anxiety among girls means that even more SSRI scripts will be written. Teenage girls are further caught in a "Catch 22", since depression is also a side effect of hormonal imbalances as well as the pill. How many females will be diagnosed with PMDD and then put on Prozac/Sarafem or one of the many SSRIs, will one day find themselves facing a breast cancer diagnosis or a suicide attempt?

A Dangerous Trend

Young women have become fair game these days by pharmaceutical companies hungry for profits. Whether it's the prescribing of the pill or antidepressants, many dangers lie in wait. Young women with hormonal imbalances are not diseased nor do they have a psychiatric problem. It is a truly dangerous trend to accept such erroneous labels.

Instead of resorting to taking a pill to mask important warning signs, our daughters, must be taught to make healthy choices through diet and lifestyle. Competent holistic health practitioners are important allies in regaining hormonal health. There are many ways to assist the body to regain hormonal health. The following modalities have successfully addressed many hormonal problems: naturopathy, oriental medicine (acupuncture and Chinese herbs), Western herbalism, clinical nutrition, homeopathy, chiropractic, osteopathy, and Auyerveda.

Even more challenging is the task of healing deeply held cultural myths. If women are truly to regain and maintain their health and appreciation for their bodies, old myths and superstitions must be exorcised from our collective unconscious. The erroneous beliefs that are held about the female anatomy are passed on from generation to generation. Unless we choose to teach them otherwise our daughters are the recipients of this legacy. By healing these misconceptions, women can truly honor and appreciate their bodies—an important prerequisite for overall hormonal balance.

A Final Word

Medicalizing and pathologizing young women's menstrual cycles and hormonal imbalances must stop. Menstrual cycles are not diseases, aberrations of nature or psychiatric conditions.

If a young woman is prescribed the pill to help correct hormonal health problems such as PMS, ovarian cysts or endometriosis, her already impaired health will only suffer further and longer. Reducing or stopping the presenting symptoms through the use of the pill is not the same thing as healing the body and regaining health. Prolonged and chronic imbalances begin to break down the body's ability to function. For some women, the effects may show up relatively soon in their life; while others may experience the consequences after years or decades. Helping young women to stay healthy by educating them about their miraculous bodies and offering them healthy alternatives goes a long way towards a lifetime of good health.

PART FIVE

Appreciating
The Female Body

Chapter 1
The Vessel Of Wisdom

The modern woman is an unstoppable force. She can run her own business, become a university dean, a politician, a doctor, or pilot an F16. Yet, ask her about how her reproductive system works or what exactly happens when she menstruates, and nine times out of ten, you'll be met with a blank stare. How is it todays women have come so far in achieving liberation and success, and still can be so lost and disconnected from the knowledge and appreciation of their own bodies and natural cycles? Women's wisdom seems to have been usurped by modern technology. At the drop of a pill, we can work hocus pocus with our hormones. Pop on a patch...and presto...periods will disappear! Is this really progress?

What happens to the nine year old girl who, after viewing TV ads for Ortho-Triclyclin, asks her mom if she will be able take the pill when she begins her period to prevent pimples? What about the teenager, who hates getting her period because of painful cramps, so she decides to take a Depo-Provera shot stopping it altogether for months?

The girls who eat their sugar coated breakfast cereal, skip lunch, drink three Diet Cokes a day, stay up late and have a frozen dinner will find it almost impossible to have a healthy, well-functioning body.

The female reproductive system is incredibly sensitive to the substances, thoughts and emotions we feed it. Hate, resist, invalidate, deny and drug our body's functions, and a downward spiral of hormonal problems, infertility, depression and disease will, all too predictably, occur. The seeds of chronic illness, like breast cancer, are sown early in a woman's life. The dietary and life style choices young girls and teenagers make ultimately, determine the quality of their life-long health. An unhealthy, toxic, stressed teenager or young woman is a candidate for PMS, endometriosis, ovarian cysts, polycystic ovaries, fibroids, painful periods or absent periods.

Without the knowledge and appreciation of the inner

workings of the female body, girls will continue to be abusive to their bodies and resort to pharmaceutical drugs to deal with the symptoms. Every drug has multiple side effects which further compromises the body's ability to function.

Once again, it is the responsibility of mothers to teach our daughters to love their bodies and all its functions. It's time to initiate our girls into the power and beauty of menstrual wisdom.

So, why are so many women oblivious to the power and healing hidden within their unique physiology? How can we help our daughters reclaim the love and appreciation of themselves as women?

A Look Back at History

History is written by the winners. Winners may be the conquering armies, political factions, religious movements or economic interests. The winners may also be prevailing belief systems, philosophies or theories. Until rather modern times, a two thousand year old attitude prevailed when it came to understanding women and their bodies.

In the ancient world, all things male were exalted. Ancient Greek anatomist and philosophers, such as Galen, firmly thought that a woman's physiology was a rather inferior copy of a male's. A woman's reproductive system was merely an inside out version of the male anatomy, the uterus was the female scrotum, the ovaries were testicles, the vulva was a foreskin and the vagina was a penis.

Medical myths throughout the centuries have generated some rather strange ideas about the female physiology. Hippocrates, the grand old man of modern medicine, obviously didn't think too highly of women. He asked the question, "What is woman?" He then proceeded to offer the answer "Disease!" He also believed the uterus was an organ wandering unfettered through a woman's' body, giving rise to any number of physical, mental and moral feelings. The word hysteria, after all, comes from the Greek word for womb. Hippocrates also believed the human uterus had as many as seven chambers and was lined with 'tentacles' or 'suckers'.

Hippocrate's blunder persisted until the Renaissance, when Leonardo da Vinci, for the first time, correctly drew the uterus and the fetus with its umbilical cord. Leonardo got it almost right. He promoted the idea a "milk vein" extended from the uterus up to the breast, to transform blood from the pregnant uterus into milk for the newborn. As recently as the nineteenth century, physicians argued the uterus competes directly with the brain for an adequate blood supply. Thus, any effort a woman made to nourish her mind through education or career could come only at the expense of her fertility. Many a school door was shut to women eager to learn.

The negative perception about menstruation also has ancient roots. Hippocrates argued fermentation in the blood precipitated menstruation because women lacked the male ability to dissipate impurities in the blood gently and sweetly through sweat. To him menstrual blood had a 'noisome smell'. Galen, another revered Greek doctor, believed menstrual blood was the residue of blood in food. Therefore, women, having smaller and inferior bodies, were unable to digest this food residue. Then there's the great philosopher Aristotle who assumed menses came from excess blood not incorporated into the fetus.

The notion menstrual blood is toxic has pervaded human thinking not only through time but also throughout the world. All kinds of strange myths were believed. Given the noxious fumes they supposedly exuded, menstruating women were thought to make meat go bad, turn wine sour, make bread dough fall and blunt knives. Menstruating women were often shunned and forced to be confined to their homes.

In the Middle Ages, just about whatever ailed a woman,

and this included non-medical 'problems' such as, sinfulness, sexuality and emotionalism, were all blamed on her reproductive organs. Two centuries later, when modern medicine was in its unscientific infancy, physicians fixated on the uterus as the source of just about every complaint a woman might voice.

The "science" of gynecology had its beginning in the mid-Victorian era when attitudes to women were, at their most bizarre, a curious mixture of contempt and idealism. Women were thought of as pale, delicate flowers who wilted easily. They required great care, even in small matters, preferably under medical supervision. Many well-meaning Victorian doctors performed hysterectomies, oopherectomies (removal of ovaries) and cliterectomies (removal of the clitoris) as legitimate treatments for resolving many of women's physical and psychological problems.

Women were also "proven" to be intellectually inferior to men. According to the popular 19th-century physician and medical philosopher, Charles Meigs, "women's heads were almost too small for intellect but just big enough for love". The prevailing theory cautioned women against developing their intellect since it would cause the uterus to atrophy! Scientific 'studies' published in 1860's demonstrated black men had smaller brains than white men and women had the smallest brains of all.

The concept of the uterus as a "dominant organ" controlling women's behavior has obsessed gynecologists for more than a century. Such conditions as hysterical mania, nymphomania, depression and even the 'uncontrollable urge to waltz' could be cured simply by removing the cause, the uterus. This left the woman passive, happy and relieved of "the cause of menstruation".

In the years following the introduction of anesthesia, a woman was likely to find herself on the operating table for just about anything her husband, father or doctor might decide was wrong with her: overeating, painful menstruation, attempted suicide, and most particularly, masturbation, erotic tendencies or promiscuity. The doctors of the day were convinced, and persuaded their patients, that a hysterectomy had a calming effect that would render women more "tractable, orderly, industrious and cleanly.

Thank goodness we now live in more enlightened times. Or do we? In 1971, the *American College of Obstetrician and Gynecologists* expressed their opinion about the uterus. In all their wisdom, they proclaimed the uterus was a "useless, bleeding, symptom producing potential cancer bearing organ."

Unfortunately, it appears women's reproductive organs are often still perceived as the source of her problems or at least compromising her physical and emotional health. To protect women, many doctors will recommend prophylactic surgery to remove perfectly healthy breasts, uteruses and ovaries. Quite often, these procedures were discovered to be totally unnecessary.

More recently the medicalization of women has focused on the prophylactic use of the pill. Major articles in *Time Magazine, The New Yorker, The Guardian* and many of the women's magazines are trumpeting yet another new reason to take the pill. The so-called "experts" have theorized that modern women are having too many menstrual cycles. They seem to be suffering from a "Period Disease". They postulate that our Stone Age sisters menstruated less frequently in their life time.

Since the 450 or so menstrual cycles a Western woman experiences in her life time are deemed unscientific, unproven and possibly even unnatural, not to mention rather messy and inconvenient, it is now highly recommended that women take a continuous low dose pill.

This new, popular fad is an unprecedented health disaster in the making. Totally unproven, this theory is gaining momentum amongst both practitioners and women, especially young women. Why worry about having your period during the prom? Taking a trip? Now you can leave your tampons at home. What about the important business meeting? Eliminate embarrassing red stains. It seems the pharmaceutical industry will stop at nothing to increase their coffers, even if it means sacrificing young women's health and fertility.

If women are to truly regain and maintain their health and love for their bodies, old myths and superstitions must be exorcised from our collective unconscious. The erroneous conscious and unconscious beliefs that are held about the female anatomy, are passed on from generation to generation. Our daughters are the recipients of this legacy unless we choose to teach them otherwise. By healing these misconceptions, women can truly honor and appreciate their bodies, a prerequisite for hormonal health and balance.

It's time to lift the veil of ignorance. The truth about a woman's physiology is nothing less, than awe-inspiring.

Many myths and misunderstandings have veiled the true function and purpose of the ovaries throughout a woman's entire life.

Hidden deep within each woman are a pair of truly amazing organs - the ovaries. They not only embody the mystery of life and the cycle of reproduction, they also hold the secrets of a woman's transformation and renewal.

The ovaries are small, oblong, pearl-colored organs lying just below the fallopian tubes at either side of the uterus. They are the size and shape of an unshelled almond, but a lumpy and irregular almond. Ovaries are scarred and pitted because each ovulation leaves behind a white blemish where an egg follicle, the sac containing the immature egg, has been emptied of its contents. The more ovulations a woman has, the more pitted the ovaries become.

They are a woman's primary sex organs. The ovaries produce the two key female hormones, progesterone and estrogen, essential in ensuring her reproductive capacities. A developing female fetus contains all of the immature eggs, known as follicles that will mature and be released during a woman's entire fertile life. The ovaries of the female fetus contain about seven million follicles! By the time puberty arrives, the number of follicles has been reduced to about 400,000 and only about 400 of them actually develop during a woman's life.

A follicle is a balloon-like sac, which holds the immature egg in a protective fluid. When an egg in residence in the ovary responds to hormonal signals from the brain, the tissue surrounding it begins to enlarge and matures into a follicle. It then moves to the outside edge of the ovary. As it enlarges, the follicle to makes estrogen that flows into the blood stream. Every month about 20 follicles are enlisted in the process of maturing eggs. Normally only one succeeds in releasing its egg before the others. This is called ovulation.

The follicle then ejects the egg into the waiting arms of the fallopian tube, the viaduct, transporting the egg to the uterus. Actually, it's really the waving fingers, the fembricel, which are covered with tiny projections, beat in sync and duide the egg along the tube to its ultimate destination, the uterus. If women have a blocked or missing fallopian tube, it is possible for an egg to make it from one ovary into the fallopian tube on the opposite side.

When it comes to fertilizing an egg, old theories really get turned on their head. Up until 1980, biology texts describing fertilization emphasized the passivity of the egg waiting for the sperm to awaken it; the way the prince's kiss awakens Sleeping Beauty. However, an electron microscope changed that theory. It was discovered the sperm does not burrow into the slumbering egg. Instead, the cell surface of the egg extends small fingerlike projections, known as the mound of microvilli, that clasp the sperm and draw it into the cell.

Although the mound of microvilli reaching toward the sperm had been observed since 1895, it had been ignored. Through research it was discovered the egg and sperm are mutually active partners. The mammalian female reproductive tract also has been viewed as passive. Now studies reveal the sperm must be capacitated by secretions from the female genital tract before it can fertilize the egg. Upon reaching the egg, the sperm releases enzymes that digest some of the extracellular vestments surrounding the egg, but these enzymes cannot function until they are activated by another secretion from the female reproductive tract.

Making eggs isn't the ovaries only function any more than reproduction is a woman's whole function. The ovary is more than just as egg sac. It's an endocrine organ - a hormone producing organ. Hormones are produced before, during and after menopause. During menopause the ovary goes through a shift from a follicle rich producer of estrogen and progesterone into a producer of estrogen and androgen. In the postmenopausal woman the ovary responds with increased production of testosterone and continues to lower levels of the estrogens, estrone and estradiol and the estrogen precursor, androstenedione.

So, contrary to popular belief, the ovaries do not shrivel up or cease functioning at menopause. Ovaries produce hormones, including estrogen, throughout life. The amounts produced will change depending on a woman's age.

Since the menopausal woman is no longer in her reproductive cycle, it is not necessary for the body to produce the
high levels of estrogen required to mature an egg. Therefore,
as women age, the ovaries grow smaller, as nature intended.
However, the part of the ovary that does shrink is known as
the theca, the outermost covering where the eggs grow and
develop. The innermost part of the ovary, known as the inner
stroma, actually becomes active for the first time in a woman's
life. With exquisite timing, one functioning starts up as the other
winds down.

Conventional medicine has also held the theory estrogen
production begins to decline during the perimenopausal years.
This is not true. Dr. Jerilynn Prior, a world renowned endocrinologist, thoroughly reviewed all pertinent references from
1990 to the present and found no evidence estrogen levels fall
before menopause. All evidence indicates over-all estrogen
production remains at normal premenopausal levels. After
menopause the ovaries continue to function, working in conjunction with other body sites, such as, the adrenal glands,
skin, muscle, brain, pineal gland, hair follicles and body fat
to produce hormones. Celso Ramon Garcia, M.D., Director of
Surgery at the University of Pennsylvania Hospital , has found
hormones produced by the postmenopausal ovaries promotes
bone health and skin suppleness, supports sexual functioning,
protects against heart disease and contribute to a woman's
health and well-being.

The ovaries have as much to do with the maintenance of
a woman's own life as they do with her role of bringing other
lives into the world.

Ovaries are not only vital physical structures of a woman's physiology, but also are expressions of her emotional and
spiritual essence. The ovarian wisdom represents a woman's
deepest creativity; the unique creative expression which waits
to be born within her. All of the creations that come from deep

within, whether they are babies, books, or works of art, have a life of their own. An important aspect of a woman's journey is to allow her creative expressions to be birthed and nurtured unfettered.

Our ability to yield to our creativity amd to acknowledge we cannot control it with our intellects, is the key to understanding ovarian power. We must allow this power to come through us.

When a woman's fears or insecurities prevent her from heeding her innermost creative wisdom, ovarian problems can arise. Ovarian dysfunction results from a woman's perception that people and circumstances outside of herself prevent her from being creative. When a woman uses her emotional weaponry to indulge in being highly critical or seeking revenge, it is often the health of her ovaries at risk.

The uterus, also known as the womb, is a remarkable and powerful muscular organ. The size of a fist in a non-pregnant woman, it can expand to the size of a watermelon in the last trimester of pregnancy. It weighs about two ounces and is roughly three inches long. By the end of pregnancy, however, it has grown to two pounds and it's volume has increase a thousandfold!!

While estrogen stimulates the growth of the uterine lining, the uterus itself does not make estrogen. This physiological fact seems to have eluded even the most erudite doctor since estrogen is routinely prescribed to women who have had a hysterectomy.

The uterus has two parts, each making up about half its length. The body, or fundus, is where the fetus develops. The cervix, projects down into the vagina and opens slightly for the release of menstrual blood and more gapingly for the birth of a baby.

The uterus is loosely held in its pelvic girdle by six ligaments. These ligaments are flexible bands of fibrous tissue offering support for the organ and enclosing the blood vessels that nourish it. The position of the uterus shifts in the pelvis depending on whether you're prone or upright and, if your bladder is full or empty.

Natalie Angier, author of *Woman: An Intimate Geography* marvels at the creation of the uterus.

> "It must be open to change, yet stable... it must be capable of growing in adulthood as no other organ grows. It must communicate with the rest of the body to discern where it is in the do-si-do between ovulation and menstruation. The uterus is a part of the endocrine system, the macrame of glands, organs and brain structures that secrete and respond to hormones. It is enmeshed biochemically with

the adrenals, the ovaries, the hypothalamus and the pituitary. At the same time it is a privileged place, a dome apart, where the fetus will not be ejected by the body's immune cells."

The uterus also is an important sex organ. The accelerating pitch of sexual excitement prompts the uterus to contract and rise out of the vagina. At orgasm, it undergoes a series of contractions. All the other so-called orgasms (vaginal, clitoral and nipple) are the initiators of sexual excitement. Uterine contractions are the end point of this excitement and female orgasm requires these contractions.

The uterus has received great homage in fertile women as the receptacle that nurtures and nourishes the developing fetus. However, as soon as menopause comes along many doctors and women believe it has fulfilled its mission in life and can now be bid a fond adieu. Nothing could be further from the truth. Far from a useless, disposable organ, the menopausal uterus is actually the site for the production of the hormone, prostacylin, which is known to protect women from heart disease and unwanted blood clotting. Since prostacylin cannot be synthetically manufactured, the removal of uterus will ensure its production will forever cease.

The uterus also serves a structural role. Like any strong foundation, it helps to keep the organs of the abdominal cavity in their place. Once removed, organs can collapse causing all sorts of problems from prolapsed organs to structural changes in the hips and length of the legs.

Breasts are one of the true marvels of nature. When you think of women, breasts will usually be the first image that pops into your mind. Breasts are intriguing, fascinating, tantalizing, seductive and one of the most alluring characteristics of the female gender. They come in all sizes and shapes; infinite varieties on a theme. Breasts are expressions not only of the aesthetic beauty of women but also their sensuality, sexuality, fertility, and nurturing. Breasts feed and sustain new life. No other organ, apart from the uterus, changes so dramatically in size, shape and function as the breast does during puberty, pregnancy and lactation.

Like many aspects of the female physiology, the breasts are superb expressions of divine creation. The origins of the breast are found in the growing fetus. Breast tissue begins to develop by the 4th week of fetal life. It grows along two parallel milk ridges, ancient mammalian structures extending from the armpits down to the groin. By the 9th week, the milk ridges regress to just the chest area. In the fetal world, both males and females have milk ridges but only in females do they receive enough hormonal stimulation later in life to blossom into breasts.

The mammary glands found in each breast, are made of specialized tissue that evolved into a modified sweat gland. Milk is actually highly enriched sweat. Prolactin, the hormone responsible for milk production, predates the evolution of mammals. It originally served to maintain salt and water balance in early vertebrates literally allowing fish to sweat.

The aesthetic breast develops in advance of the glandular one. Early in adolescent the brain begins secreting regular bursts of hormones to stimulate the ovaries. The ovaries, in turn, discharge estrogen and estrogen encourages the body to lay down fat deposits in the breast. The adipose tissue is suspended in a gelatinous matrix of connective fibers extending from the muscle of the chest wall to the underside of the breast skin. It is seldom realized how extensively breast tissue is distributed, reaching from the collarbone down to the last two ribs and from the breastbone in the middle of the chest to the back of the armpits. The lymph system serves a most important function as the body's garbage disposal system. It is an important part of the body's immune system. This is a system of organs, including the spleen, the thymus, the tonsils and the lymph nodes. A clear fluid called lymph circulates through the lymphatic vessels in the body. The lymph also bathes the body's cells. The lymphatic system provides a continuous cleansing and operates on the cellular levels.

The lymph nodes and tubes carry white blood cells, called lymphocytes, cleaning the breasts of waste products, impurities, viruses, infections and cancer cells. The lymph system is densely interwoven into the breast tissue. The lymph nodes under the arm (the axillary lymph nodes) are usually those involved first in breast cancer. Doing a gently lymphatic massage all around the breast area on a regular basis is an effective way to assist lymphatic drainage.

Connective tissue has the unique ability to stretch and can accommodate as much fat as the body inserts between its fibers. It's the connective tissue that gives breasts their bounce. While estrogen is necessary for breast development, it is not the only factor explaining the wide variability in breast size. A woman who develops large breasts doesn't necessarily have higher estrogen levels than a small-breasted woman. Rather, it is the breast tissue's responsiveness to estrogen stimulation. A woman's sensitivity is determined, in part, by genetic make-up. Among sensitive women, a very small amount of estrogen fosters a generous bosom. Estrogen sensitive women who take the birth control pill, which has high levels of estrogen, discover their breasts increase in size.

Other hormonal influences also hold sway over the breasts. Thyroid hormones, stress hormones, growth hormones and insulin all have an effect on breast development.

The hormone estrogen gives the areola a subtly darker color.

Estrogen also spurs the development of the glandular tissue that will one day secrete milk. A series of firm, rubbery ducts or pathways and lobes begin threading their way through the fat, connective tissue, blood vessels and nerves of the breast. Each breast usually ends up with between 15-20 lobes, or milk glands. Each lobe has its independent duct, the carrying milk to the nipple. The lobes are divided into about two dozen lobules, which look like tiny clusters of grapes.

While the lobes and lobules are distributed fairly evenly throughout the breast, the ducts lead to a single destination, the nipple. As the ducts converge on the nipple, curling and bending, their diameter widens. The lobes and lobules are like the foliage, the fruits and the leaves of a tree while the ducts are the branches thickening into a braid of trunks. Milk is generated in each tiny lobular fruit and pulsed to the spacious pipeline below. The ducts perforate the skin of the nipple. When a woman is nursing , her nipples balloon out and look like a watering can, each ductal hole visible and visibly secreting milk.

The ducts, lobes and lobulars do not fully mature until pregnancy when they proliferative, thicken and differentiate.

In Western cultures the usual age for the beginning of breast growth use to be around 11 or 12, old. Now that is changing.

Girls as young as eight, or even younger, are now showing signs of breast development. In most girls the non-fatty breast tissue is developed by the age 15 or 16. Fat makes up about 13 percent of breast tissue. The breasts can grow or shrink with weight loss or gain.

In the puberty cycle, pubic hair usually begins to grow first. Only after pubic hair has made its presence does the breast begin to awaken. Breast tissue starts to respond to the hormonal changes occurring in a young girl's body. Typically, it takes a year or two after the breast begins developing for the menses to start. Breast development begins with a little bud of breast tissue under the nipple. As the tissue begins responding to the hormonal stimulation, the tiny breast buds can itch and may become somewhat painful. The rudimentary ducts begin to grow and the breast expands more and more until they reach their full growth, usually by the time of a girl's first period.

Given the significant percentage of fatty tissue in breasts, they are adversely affected by environmental toxins such as pesticides , industrial waste and heavy metals. All of these potentially damaging ingredients tend to be stored in fat, especially in breast fat. As long as a toxin is in fatty tissue, it poises a serious threat to the health and genetic integrity of the cells of nearby lobules and ducts. The presence of these toxins creates a very dangerous game of breast cancer Russian roulette.

Sat Dharam Kaur N.D., author of *A Call to Women* is worried about the risk to the tree-like inner physiology of the mammary glands. " I think of this 'tree' in our breasts as being a hidden tree of life. Breast milk is the fruit. Normally breast milk sustains life. Today, chemical pollutants and radiation poison the fruit, just as our air, water, soil and many planetary life forms are poisoned. The breast cancer epidemic is a but a symptom and symbol of our plant in crises and of the poisoned and dying tree of life."

There's no doubt about it. The nurturing, sexy, sensual breasts of young women are extremely vulnerable to the many dangers lurking in our twenty first century world.

Each month a ritual repeats itself. The lining of the uterus thickens in preparation for the implantation of a fetus and, if none, arrives, it is shed. Menstruation is the ultimate expression of what it is to be female. It means surrendering to the body's natural rhythms, to the flow of life that goes on within us and beyond conscious control. It is really a wonder.

The origin of the word "menstruation" has long been associated with power. The power is present even in the word menstruation. In the earliest cultures, it meant "incomprehensible", "supernatural", "spirit" and "deity". In German, French, and Spanish, the word menstruation also means "measure" or "rule" and connects with the terms "regulate, regal, regalia and rex (king).

The word "blessing" originates from the old English "bloodsen" which means bleeding. In Celtic Britain, claret was the traditional drink of kings. It was also a synonym for blood, and literally meant "enlightenment". According to the Taoist tradition in China, a man could become immortal if he absorbed menstrual blood, called red yin juice, from a woman's Mysterious Gateway. The significance and power of menstruation resonates loud and clear in many cultures and throughout the ages.

What exactly happens to the uterus at menstruation? The cervix and fundus are both composed of three layers of tissue types. The meat in the middle is the thick myometrium, and consists of three interwrapping sheets of muscle. On the outside of the myometrium is a thick covering, the serous membrane, which is similar in texture and function to the sacs surrounding the heart and lungs. Like those sacs, the uterine serous membrane keeps the organ wet and cushioned.

On the other side of the myometrium is the uterine lining, the endometrium. The endometrium is made of three layers of mucous membrane. Unlike serous membranes, the mucous membrane breathes and secretes. It absorbs waters, salts and other compounds. It releases mucus, a mixture of white blood cells, water, the sticky protein known as mucin, and cast-off tissue cells. Menstruation is in part, a mucus discharge. During menstruation, two of the mucous sheaths are shed. They are then recreated when the cycle begins anew. The third, deepest layer does not shed but, instead, becomes the stable foundation for a potential placenta.

Western women usually menstruate 450-480 times in their lifetime. During the average period, about six tablespoons, or three ounces, of material is cast off. Half of it is blood and the other half is the shedding endometrial layers, along with vaginal and cervical secretions.

The actual mechanism of menstruation is a truly brilliant design. Feeding into the two disposable layers of the endometrium are three spiral arteries, resembling corkscrews. Several days before menstruation begins, the tips of the spirals grow longer and more tightly coiled. It's as though they're being pulled and twisted at the same time. Circulation to the endometrium grows sluggish. Twenty-four hours before the onset of bleeding, the spiral artery constricts sharply and the blood flow ceases. Deprived of blood and oxygen, the endometrial tissue dies. Then, as abruptly as the arteries squeezed shut, they temporarily open again, allowing blood to rush in. The blood pools in pockets beneath the dead endometrium, causing the lining to swell and burst, thus initiating a period. Then the spiral arteries constrict once again. (Fibroids disturb the ritual of menstruation because their parasitic blood supply does not conform to the squeeze-relax-squeeze, pattern of the spiral arteries.)

Another feature of menstruation is the blood, itself. Most blood is poised to clot. The blood flows briefly and then coagulates. However, menstrual blood does not clot. It may thicken at times, and the dead tissues accompanying it may pass out in clots , but it does not behave as normal blood. The only reason menstrual blood does not keep flowing is that the spiral arteries constrict in the wake of endometrial death.

Each month a woman recapitulates the phases of creation, nourishment, death and regeneration. The changes occurring each month are not only physiological. A woman's emotional and mental self is expressed in this ebb and flow. From the first day of menstruation until ovulation is known as the follicular phase. During this time, a woman's "creavity" can be used to conceive artistic and intellectual offspring as well as actual children. The premenstrual phase of the cycle is frequently accompanied by heightened activity, intellectual clarity, and feelings of well-being, happiness and sexual desire.

If pregnancy does not occur, the second half of the cycle is known as the luteal phase - from ovulation until the onset of menstruation. This is when there is a desire to retreat from outer activities into a more reflective mode. The inner space nurtures the opportunity to develop or "give birth" to something that comes from deep inside. This is the time women are most in tune with their inner knowing and understanding of what isn't working in their lives.

Premenstrually, the "veil between worlds" of the seen and unseen, the conscious and unconscious, is much thinner. It is when intuitive wisdom is the strongest and dreams most revealing. Access to parts of the self are off limits at other times of the month. This is when a woman can enter into her power; the ability to change things for the better because they are able to connect with and be guided by their inner self.

Women, must again reclaim the great wisdom inherent in the monthly cyclic nature of their menstruation instead of holding the perception that it is a "curse", a time of suffering, embarrassment and shame? In Native American culture, menstruation was a woman's time of power because she was able to enter an expanded reality.

Alexandra Pope, an Australian psychotherapist, author and teacher of menstrual wisdom explains how menstruation is power.

"The stress sensitive barometer in women, the menstrual cycle is an exquisite system for sensing both physical and psychological well-being. Menstruation is an initiatory time, when women can potentially open to a highly charged altered state, giving them access to a singular kind of power. The power of self-awareness, deep feeling, knowingness, intuition. A power that matures over time with each cycle.

Cycles are the very basis of life, the means by which nature and humans regenerate. To go against them is a recipe for disaster. To listen to them adds a richness and connection to life. Women who medicate their menstrual cycle are in danger not only of harming their physical health, but also of cauterizing the depths of their inner natures. Something will never feel complete. In short, they can end up living a half life.

The tendencies in the ovulatory phase of the cycle are more outer focused, linear, left brain, feeling fairly clear (no messy emotion) and pro-ductive, with plenty of energy for others. As we move into the menstrual phase of the cycle women tend to become more inner focused. The transition to this inner state is often signaled by feelings of irritability, anger, overwhelm, greater dreaminess and vagueness. The people around us often feel more like an irritant.

Opposites are amplified. For example you may experience feeling driven one moment and then flip into its opposite, becoming drifty and dreamy the next. A feeling of purposefulness may fall away to be replaced by questioning about one's self and what one is doing. This can also take the form of criticism of self and others, or simply depression. The single most dominant characteristic of this phase is sensitivity. We become more permeable both to our own depths and to the world.

Sensitivity is a wonderful opening to feeling and spirit. If you can travel through this opening with greater acceptance, you'll experience an illumination and knowingness for the whole of your life. Your deep feelings are an awesome intelligence, a form of knowing beyond surface realities. Without our capacity for depth of feeling, and, yes, it includes all the so-called 'negative' ones; life would lack meaning and intimacy, ecstasy and joy.

The sensitivity extends the acreage of our souls, encourages us to examine and challenge ourselves and the world we live in. If the task feels too great, the sensitivity of menstruation too overwhelming, we should neither condemn menstruation nor ourselves. It would be like shooting the messenger. We must learn to value and harness the power that comes from our greater openness. Take a stand for more womanly ways of knowing. Track your feelings, listen to gut instincts, notice synchronicities, catch the intuitive flashes and recognize the connections between all things. Intellect is immeasurably matured by such skills of knowing.

Menstruation is the call to attend to ourselves and to matters beyond the mundane surface level of existence. True power comes from our capacity to travel in both inner and outer worlds, to experience emotional and spiritual depths along with our intellectual rigor. This is true for both women and men. Women are blessed with an inner process, the menstrual cycle. This is a wonderful gift and truly a blessing."

A Native American saying proclaims, "At menarche a young woman enters her power, throughout her menstruating years she practices her power and at menopause she becomes her power." Every stage of a woman's life cycle offers an opportunity for her to reach into the wellspring of wisdom. Ignore it or be oblivious to it, and it is lost.

As mothers reclaim the power, beauty and great wisdom that sculpted the female physiology, they can pass on to generations of daughters a healing legacy of love, respect and power for the female body and spirit.

PART SIX

Creating A Healthy Body And Balanced Hormones

Forewarned is forearmed, as the saying goes. This is particularly true in knowing exactly what's going on with our hormones. The solutions are straightforward when the problem is clearly understood. This is a really tall order when it comes to understanding the nature of our endocrine system and the hormones it makes. Why? Because so much of the information women are given about their body and how it works is seriously tainted by myths, misinformation or down right lies. As always, getting the story straight will go a long way to empowering mothers to make the best possible choices for their daughters and themselves. So, let's have a lesson about hormones.

Hormones regulate all systems of the body. They are organic compounds secreted by the various cells, tissues, organs and the endocrine system. The hormones our body makes are usually short lived, staying in the blood stream for just a few minutes, at most a few hours. After a hormonal message is delivered, the liver breaks it down and either flushes it out of the body or recycles it to build other molecules

The endocrine system, responsible for sending out hormonal signals, includes nine glands: hypothalamus, pineal, pituitary, thyroid, parathyroid, thymus, adrenals, pancreas, and ovaries. These ductless endocrine glands send small amounts of hormones, which carry important messages throughout the body. Besides these glands, the endocrine system also includes pockets of hormone-producing cells in tissues residing in the small intestine, heart, kidneys and stomach. By the end of the second trimester of fetal development, the fetus' endocrine system begins producing hormones.

Although very small in size, hormones pack a very big wallop. They are measured in teeny, tiny amounts – in parts per billion and parts per trillion. Progesterone, for instance, is measured in parts per billion; estrogen works in parts trillion.

The smallest amounts of these hormones create powerful changes in the body.

This is a simplified explanation of how hormones work:

"The hormone jumps on its trusty bicycle and rides through the blood stream until it finds the correct address - the cells of a specific organ or tissue meant to receive the message. The hormone finds a place to park, called a receptor, located either at the cell surface or inside the cell, and delivers a message. The signal has been delivered from one cell to another.

Now there is a response. Central headquarters in the cell takes the message and runs with it. The message is copied and translated into orders, which are sent to various parts of the body. For example, the pituitary is an endocrine gland sends signals to the ovary, which then sends e-mail messages to the uterus and in response, the uterus sheds its lining.[1]"

However, hormone disrupting chemicals can cause signals to go awry. An unnatural signal may create an inappropriate response. Science has now discovered hormone disruptors can bind with receptors and send messages in the same way our natural hormones can. The problem is that these messages give faulty instructions.

The word estrogen is not the name of any specific hormone but rather a classification for a large group of compounds with estrogenic properties. These include all kinds of estrogens: human, animal, synthetic, phytoestrogens and xenoestrogens. The three major human estrogens are estradiol, estrone and estriol. Estradiol is 1000 times more potent in its effects on breast tissue than estriol, the weakest estrogen. Estradiol is the predominant estrogen during a woman's reproductive stage of life; estrone is a dominant hormone postmenopausally; and estriol is abundant during pregnancy. The body can convert estradiol to estrone and vice versa.

The ovaries begin to produce estrogen during puberty, usually anywhere between 10 and 14 years of age. During a single menstrual cycle, the ovaries produce increasing amounts of estrogen from the first day of the period leading up to the day of ovulation in an effort to prepare the uterus for a possible pregnancy. Estrogen levels peak just before ovulation. After ovulation, estrogen levels drop for a few days and then increase less dramatically until the end of the menstrual cycle.

One of estrogen's jobs is to make cells multiply. Estrogen's message to the cells is "grow, grow, grow". It is this female hormone which produces secondary sex characteristics in women. We have estrogen to thank for the curvy hips and the developing of breasts during puberty. It is estrogen's tendency to stimulate cell growth making its excess such a dangerous promoter of cancer when it is out of balance

Estrogen's effects are also seen on the ovaries, cervix, fallopian tubes, vagina, external genitalia and breasts. It is also necessary for the maintenance of menstrual cycles and pregnancy, specifically creating the uterus' blood-rich lining necessary for the implantation of a fetus. Vocal cord changes are also attributable to estrogen. The emergence of estrogen at puberty stops the growth of long bones in both males and females. Just prior to puberty there is a spurt in height and after puberty, when estrogen is higher, height does not increase.

It was once thought estrogen would bind mainly with estrogen receptors in the female organs. It is now known there are estrogen receptors lining the blood vessels, in the brain, bones, liver, kidneys, adrenals and eyes. So estrogen has an affect throughout the body.

Progesterone is often considered estrogen's stepchild when hormones are discussed.

Unlike estrogen, progesterone is not a classification of hormones but rather a specific hormone produced by the corpus luteum after ovulation and, in smaller quantities, by the adrenal glands. It is also a precursor hormone, which means other hormones such as testosterone, estrogen and corticosteroids are made from it. During pregnancy, the placenta makes copious amounts of it.

Progesterone, like estrogen, affects every tissue in your body including the breasts, uterus, brain cells, fat metabolism, water balance, bone cells, and development of the fetus. Like testosterone, it is an anabolic steroid, helping to build tissue, creating energy and furthering the growth and repair of the body. Progesterone does not confer secondary sex characteristics.

Progesterone is made the second half of a woman's menstrual cycle. When an egg is released, ovulation, the follicle, the sac holding the egg, transforms into the corpus luteum and produces progesterone. Progesterone is the dominant hormone during this second part of the cycle. If for some reason ovulation does not occur, progesterone is not made, and estrogen becomes the dominant hormone during the entire length of the menstrual cycle.

One of progesterone's most important and powerful functions in the body is to balance or oppose estrogen. The body works with checks and balances in an attempt to maintain homeostasis. Progesterone's role is to protect the body from estrogen's enthusiastic "grow" message. While, estrogen is responsible for the growth or proliferation of tissue, progesterone is linked to the maturation of tissue. The effect of too much estrogen is like speeding along with your foot on the accelerator; progesterone is like applying the brakes and staying within the legal speed limit!

A woman with low progesterone is more likely to be diagnosed with breast cancer than a woman with normal levels. Low progesterone may also lead to menstrual irregularities, PMS, endometriosis, ovarian cysts, depression, infertility or miscarriage. Women with low progesterone have a tenfold increase in all cancers and experience 5.4 times more breast cancer than women with normal progesterone levels.[5] One study found progesterone caused a 90 percent inhibition of cell growth in breast cancer cells, in a laboratory setting when the cells were progesterone receptor positive. This study showed when cancer cells were exposed to equivalent amounts of progesterone, as would be made in the third trimester of pregnancy, 48 percent of the cells had undergone self-destruction and another 40 percent showed signs of disintegration. Progesterone had no effect on breast cancer cell receptors. This study seems to indicate progesterone might be a powerful hormonal treatment for progesterone receptor positive breast cancer.[6]

A number of hormone disruptors inhibit progesterone. Animal studies in primates show some environmental estrogens suppress progesterone synthesis. Also, a high level of estrogen in the body can make xenoestrogens bind to progesterone receptors and plug up the receptors, preventing natural progesterone from sending its message. Thus, if some hormone disruptors inhibit progesterone, the overall trend appears to be heavily weighted toward more estrogenic signaling

Naturopath and breast cancer specialist, Sat Dharam Kaur, is concerned about the increase of low progesterone levels. "I'm regularly seeing PMS symptoms and breast swelling in women before periods which is indicative of low progesterone levels. When I check saliva levels between days 20-24 progesterone should be the highest, the women with the most PMS symptoms had the lowest progesterone levels. Pesticides and environmental chemical decrease progesterone or decrease the ability of progesterone to bind to receptor sites."

Estrogen dominance is a term first coined by physician and author, Dr. John Lee. For more than two decades, Dr. Lee has been exploring the basis for the proliferation of such female problems as PMS, endometriosis, ovarian cysts, fibroids, breast cancer, infertility, osteoporosis and menopausal problems. From his clinical experience and research, Dr. Lee discovered a consistent theme running through women's most frequent complains-too much estrogen in relationship to progesterone. The scale is heavily weighed toward the estrogen side of the hormone equation.

Again the old culprits of stress, nutritional deficiencies, a junk food diet, estrogenic substances from our environment and the use of synthetic hormones are the main factors contributing to the an estrogen dominant condition. Estrogen dominance occurs in women of all ages.

Symptoms and conditions associated with estrogen dominance

Acceleration of the aging process
Anxiety, often with depression
Autoimmune disorders such as lupus erythermatosus
and Hashimoto's thyroiditis
Breast cancer
Breast tenderness
Cervical dysplasia
Copper excess and zinc deficiency
Decreased sex drive
Depression and anxiety or agitation
Dry eyes
Early onset menstruation
Endometrial (uterine) cancer
Fat gain, especially around the hips and thighs
Fatigue

Fibrocystic breast disease
Gallbladder disease
Headaches
Hypoglycemia
Increased blood clotting/infertility
Irregular menstrual periods
Irritability
Insomnia
Magnesium deficiency
Mood swings
Osteoporosis
Polycystic ovaries
Premenopausal bone loss
PMS
Prostate cancer
Sluggish metabolism
Thyroid dysfunction mimicking hypothyroidism
Uterine cancer
Uterine fibroids
Water retention

Estrogen dominance is now a regular occurrence in young women. This is generally due to a lack of ovulation which is called an anovulatory cycle. Remember - no ovulation, no progesterone!

According to Dr. John Lee, anovulation can contribute to many hormonal health problems in women:

> "Anovulation is usually associated with low estrogen and low progesterone. During her teen years, again in her mid-thirties and forties, a woman may not ovulate during some of her monthly menstrual cycles. If you don't ovulate, you won't make progesterone in any significant amount. You can

still have a seemingly normal menstrual cycle even if you haven't ovulated but the lack of progesterone may cause you to experience PMS symptoms such as swollen and tender breasts, weight gain, mood swings and cramps. Low progesterone production tends to occur during two phases of a woman's life - at puberty and again at perimenopause. During both of these times of transition in a woman's life, her risk of breast cancer is higher. Teenagers undeveloped breast tissue is more susceptible to the growth-promoting effects of estrogen. Without the balancing effect of progesterone, estrogen has the potential to initiate or promote cancer.

Xenoestrogens exposure during embryo life damages ovarian follicles and leads to follicle failure later in life. This is a primary cause of luteal failure in premenopausal women. The near epidemic of infertility among young women today is most likely due to damage sustained by the ovaries from pollutants while they were in the womb. This type of exposure and its effect on a woman's reproductive organs causes not only infertility but also chronic estrogen dominance. Over time this will create PMS, fibrocystic breasts, fibroids, irregular periods, and endometriosis. These conditions also provide a fertile environment for estrogens to damage breast cells which can eventually lead to breast cancer."[7]

Estrogen dominance is at the very heart of most breast cancers.

Causes of Estrogen Dominance

Recently I was privileged to spend a day visiting a breast cancer center. The radiologist interpreted the mammogram x-rays while viewing them through the light box. As he explained what I was looking at, the various shadowy forms on the x-ray began to reveal their meaning. I was awed by the years of training required by radiologists to accurately decipher the x-rays illuminated before them. I was not only learning about the world of mammograms, but was also invited to accompany the doctor into the examining room, and observe as ultra sounds were taken and breast cysts aspirated Needless to say, it was a very busy center.

Talking with the radiologist and his staff of dedicated technicians, the role of estrogen in causing breast cancer came up again and again. In fact, the physician in charge of the center said, "Estrogen is my enemy." When I spoke with the women in the examining room, most were there because of having found a lump. Many of them had been taking the pill or HRT. The women were as young as 29 years old. There is no denying estrogen initiates and promotes breast cancer.

It is becoming more and more common to diagnose women in their thirties, twenties or even while in their teens with breast cancer. These younger women are often diagnosed with a more aggressive form of breast cancer. Early exposure to estrogen is a major factor. We really can't hide behind the theory of the breast cancer gene since it only affects 5-10 per-cent of all breast cancers. Obviously, something else is going on.

Known causes contributing to estrogen dominance are:

1. Birth control pills, injections and implants
2. Premarin
3. Fertility drugs – another form of estrogen
4. Anovulatory cycles
5. Exposure to environmental hormone disruptors
6. Hysterectomy
7. Being overweight
8. Overeating
9. Stress
10. Sugar
11. Candida
12. Faulty liver metabolism
13. Poor digestion and lack of healthy gut flora
14. Commercial personal care products

From this long list, it is imperative and that we detoxify our bodies, support healthy functioning of all our systems, become hormonally balanced and eliminate toxins from our personal spaces. All of this is predicated upon being educated, informed, proactive and willing to actually make the changes.

Creating and maintaining good health must become our primary goal. The principles of good health really should be taught to children from kindergarten onwards. Unfortunately, this is rarely the case.

Without the knowledge of the proper feeding and caring of your truly awesome bodies, how can you ever hope to have ongoing health? Unless you have a road map when exploring new territories, you will probably take a really long time to arrive at your destination, if you get there at all! When it comes to our collective health, it appears most of us have gotten well and truly lost!

According to the *World Health Organization*, the United States ranks thirty-seventh in overall health quality. In fact, over 75 percent of Americans are suffering from deficiency and degenerative diseases.

Young people should be expressions of vitality and health, right? Not in most western societies these days.

In 1996, the *Journal of the American Medical Association* documented 25 percent of Americans less than 18 years old had at least one chronic disease. Autopsies on adolescent accident victims in Los Angeles revealed that 80 percent had early stages of heart disease; 15 percent had arteries that were more than half blocked.

Studies are also revealing a staggering 50 percent of newly diagnosed cases of diabetes were in people under the age of nineteen. Asthma is increasing in children at an alarming rate. One of five teenagers is overweight. Teenagers are also developing significant bone loss and periodontal disease. In truth, the health of our children is in rapid and unprecedented decline.

The statistics are also equally shocking when it comes to women's hormonal imbalances. It is estimated 90 percent of women suffer from PMS. The rates of other female problems are all on the rise.

It is now estimated 5 to 10 million women suffer from endometriosis. In the beginning of the twentieth century, only 21 cases were diagnosed. Recent statistics found 15 percent of young women have Polycystic Ovarian Syndrome. The number of infertile women in the U.S. has increased to 6.1 million.

Hormonal imbalances and diseases are not random events. Rather than a game of chance, health is a choice. When imbalances occur, we can choose to address the underlying problems and resolve the problem. The trick is knowing what's going on in the body and what to do about it.

Demystifying disease requires a rudimentary understanding of the building blocks of health. It is equally true for reclaiming hormonal balance. We must learn the fundamentals of our physiology in order to get our hormones back on track. Getting to the root cause of the problem is the only way to ensure long term health.

There is a mistaken belief hormones are somehow disconnected from the rest of our body. Women often believe PMS just happens and it's part of being a woman. Rarely is it explained PMS reflects what's happening in our body i.e., our nutritional status, the health of our digestive system, our adrenals, thyroid, liver and blood sugar levels, etc.

We once thought we are what we eat. In reality it is more accurate to say we are what we digest. No matter how nutritious the food, if our digestive system is impaired, all those nutritious goodies will never make it to their final destination – building blocks for healthy cellular function.

All healing traditions believe a healthy digestive and gastrointestinal system are the keys to optimal health. Good digestion is a foundation for achieving peak performance and optimal health. Most digestive problems are the direct result of poor diets, toxic exposure, lack of exercise, unresolved stress and over-the-counter and prescription drugs.

Digestive problems may take the form of indigestion, allergic reactions to certain food, intestinal cramps, abdominal bloating, excess gas, diarrhea, constipation, low energy or difficulty concentrating and thinking. If you are not properly digesting and assimilating your foods, you will not be able to absorb vitamins and minerals, no matter how nutritious your food may be.

Proper digestion depends on the proper secretion of digestive enzymes and the digestive system's ability to assimilate and absorb foods. Most health problems begin here. No matter what foods are eaten, everything in our diets are composed of proteins, carbohydrates and fat, sugars, and fiber. The essential digestive enzymes (protease, amylase, lipase, disaccharidase and cellulase) are necessary to break down food during digestion. Without adequate enzymes, people become intolerant to certain foods, which leads to a whole host of food allergies. When enzyme deficiency is left untreated, serious health problems inevitably result.

Enzyme deficiencies include:

Compromised immune system
Chronic infections

Hormonal imbalances,
Fluid retention
Chronic constipation
Hypoglycemia
Moodiness
Depression
Irritability
Anxiety
Blood clots
Allergic reactions
Diabetes
High cholesterol
High blood pressure
Varicose veins
Impaired bone metabolism

Our modern day diet and life style contribute to the depletion of digestive enzymes. Enzymes are destroyed by pesticides and chemicals, food irradiation, hydrogenated oils, microwave cooking, radiation, fluoridation, and heavy metals such as mercury. Supplementing each meal with plant-based digestive enzymes is becoming necessity for people of all ages.

Our digestive system is residence to over 400 types of gut flora, or bacteria. These gut flora are really the hard workers that break down food into essential components for the healthy functioning of all our cells. A total of one hundred trillion bacteria live together in our digestive system, in either symbiotic or antagonist relationships. Their total weight is as much as 4 pounds. In fact, there is more bacteria in our intestinal tract than all the cells in our body!

When in balance, friendly flora is an important part of our immune system. They manufacture many vitamins including all the B vitamins, plus vitamin A and K. They also increase the bioavailability of minerals, increase our resistance to food poisoning, produce acids to keep the proper pH of the intestines, help regulate peristalsis and bowel movements, and digest proteins to free amino acids. Another important job of good gut flora is to enhance immune function. Gut flora establishes good digestion in infants, preventing colic, diaper rash and gas.

Anything interfering with the digestion of food and absorption of nutrients will compromise all aspects of our health. The worst offenders for damaging the gut flora are antibiotics, birth control pills and non-steroidal anti-inflammatory drugs like ibuprofen.

Antibiotics kill friendly bacteria and result in candida, a yeast overgrowth. Candida is a serious health problem, affecting more women than men. Candida not only has the ability to penetrate the lining of the intestine, but also release toxins and incompletely digested food and fecal matter into the blood stream. This damages the digestive tract and causes food insensitivities, allergies and other problems. Candida has been found to produce 79 different toxins, and to wreak havoc with the immune system.

Birth control pills create chemical imbalances in the gut and encouraging yeast infections. They also increase the levels of sugar present in vaginal secretions, promoting further yeast infections. Candida changes the environment in the digestive system, stimulates estrogen production and compromises the immune system.

Candida overgrowth is associated with a long list of side effects. Common problems are depression, anxiety, mood swings, lack of concentration, drowsiness, poor memory, headaches, insomnia, loss of libido, infertility, fatigue, bloating, constipation, bladder infections, menstrual cramps, vaginal itching, muscle and joint swelling, pain, hypothroidism, and skin problems.

Since candida feeds on sugar, it is important to eliminate

all forms of sugar from your diet. In fact, sugar cravings are a sign of a candida overgrowth. Anti-fungal medications are required, along with anti-fungal remedies such as grapefruit seed extract, oregano oil, coconut oil, probiotics and cultured foods.

The adrenal glands are two small prune-shaped glands that sit on top of the kidneys. Although small in size, they are very big in function. They manufacture 28 different hormones, and the digestion of food, especially carbohydrates and sugar, regulate the body's minerals, produce and maintain the body's energy levels in conjunction with the thyroid, and make hormones that monitor stress. Progesterone is the primary raw material for producing adrenal gland hormones.

Prolonged stress, whether as a result of emotional, environmental or physical causes, is disastrous for the adrenals. Initially it increases the output of the adrenal hormone, cortisol. Cortisol helps to regulate blood sugar, the movement of carbohydrates, proteins and fats in and out of the cells, reduce inflammation, and support muscle function. Long term stress causes chronically elevated levels of cortisol, result in weight gain (specially around the midsection), blood sugar imbalances, thinning skin, muscle wasting, memory loss, high blood pressure, dizziness, hot flashes, excessive facial hair, and other masculinizing tendencies.

Overworked adrenals will eventually crash leading to adrenal exhaustion and the inability to maintain adequate production of adrenal hormones.

Symptoms of overtaxed adrenals include:

Addictions to either sweet or salty foods
Allergies
Anxiety
Chronic low blood pressure
Depression
Diabetes
Extreme fatigue
Headaches

Inability to concentrate
Insomnia
Irritability
Nervousness,
Night sweats
Panic attacks
PMS
Sensitivity to cold

Do you crave salty foods such as chips, pretzels or olives? When you crave salty or sweet foods, you can be sure your adrenals are overworked. Adrenals are in charge of keeping salt and glucose levels balanced.

When the adrenals become really overwhelmed and worn out due to overeating of sweets and starches they are less able to help you with illness, trauma, injury and, of course, stress. No wonder adrenal exhaustion is such a big problem these days.

Adrenal exhaustion creates havoc with the endocrine system. Progesterone is the raw material that makes stress hormones. When the adrenal glands are in overdrive , the body will divert progesterone to the adrenals so they can continue to manufacture cortisol. Without adequate progesterone to balance estrogen in the body, an estrogen dominant condition ensues. The stress hormone, cortisol, also contributes to estrogen excess by blocking progesterone receptors.

Teenagers' obsession with weight and dieting can have life long consequences to their adrenals, affecting their hormones, moods, energy, memory, bone mass and immune systems. A study examining the role of eating attitudes in adolescent girls between the ages of 9 and 12 years found girls who were most worried about gaining weight but had not actually dieted, had a 3-5 percent lower bone mass. This disturbing trend was noted at the beginning and end of the study, two years later.

The importance of this study revealed chronic stress from just worrying about gaining weight affected the adrenals glands. Obsessing about food may prevent optimal gain of bone mass during adolescence. Overtaxed adrenal glands can result in hypothyoidism. The thyroid, the gland regulating metabolism, may turn down its hormonal activity in an attempt to reverse the adrenal overdrive. Some of the symptoms of sluggish thyroid include fatigue, weight gain, hormonal problems and depression.

Nutrients important to the adrenal glands are the B vitamins (especially B5), vitamin C, (500 mg four times a day) vitamin E, proteins, magnesium, manganese, zinc, potassium, plant enzymes, adrenal extracts, and the amino acid, tyrosine and l-theanine. Adrenal restoring herbs include licorice, maca and rhodiola rosea.

Rest is absolutely vital when it comes to rebuilding the adrenals and so is stress reduction. It is essential to get adequate sleep. Getting to bed by 10 pm is a great support for adrenal health.

The thyroid gland is an important component of the immune system. It is a small butterfly-shaped endocrine organ at the base of the neck. The thyroid is the body's thermostat and controls body temperature, energy use, the rate organs function and the speed at which the body uses food. The thyroid is implicated in the functioning of all body processes and organs. All tissues in the body are stimulated by the thyroid.

When it comes to hormonal health, the thyroid is a major player since it stimulates and synchronizes all metabolic cellular functions. The thyroid hormone is required to convert cholesterol into the vital anti-aging steroid hormones, pregnenolone, progesterone and DHEA. Pregnenolone converts to progesterone and DHEA in the body. Progesterone and DHEA are precursors for more specialized hormones, including estrogen, testosterone, and cortisol. When the thyroid hormone is inadequate, the entire hormonal system is out of kilter.

Thyroid problems are also of epidemic proportion in women - 15 to 20 times more prevalent than in men. It is estimated between 50-80 percent of western women suffer from hypothyroidism, an underactive thyroid. Hypothyroidism has a direct effect on women's hormonal health.

Conditions due to hypothyroidism

> Anxiety
> Brittle nails
> Cold hands and feet
> Constipation
> Depression
> Endometriosis
> Fatigue
> Fibrocystic breast disease
> Fibroids
> High cholesterol

Infertility
Lack of concentration
Loss of memory
Low libido
Menopausal symptoms
Migraines
Miscarriages
Muscle aches
Ovarian cysts
Poor vision
PMS
Skin problems (itching, eczema, acne, scaly)
Susceptibility to recurring infections
Swelling of eyelids
Weakened the immune system
Weight gain

Hypothyroidism studies dating back to 1950's indicate low thyroid function predisposes women to breast cancer. All hormones are intimately connected. If thyroid is low, cortisol and sex hormone production lags. Estrogen inhibits hormone activity which worsens thyroid deficiency. Hypothyroidism occurs predominately in women when estrogen is dominant and progesterone is low. Persistent estrogen dominance creates a cycle of lowered thyroid function. When the thyroid is low, estrogen is unable to activate proper amounts of a protein which binds to estrogen. Without this binding, more estrogen enters the in the blood stream and stimulate estrogen sensitive tissues.

Progesterone plays an important role in helping to maintain a healthy thyroid. In women, adequate binding of T3 , the major thyroid hormone, is dependent upon sufficient progesterone. So low levels of progesterone can predispose women to hypothyroidism. Many women with PMS and infertility, have low progesterone levels but are also hypothyroid. Also, estrogen excess interfers with the uptake of thyroid hormones also contributing to a sluggish thyroid.

We live in a thyroid toxic culture and environment. No wonder hypothyroidism is such a common disorder. Fortunately, there are very effective natural approaches to help in regulating the thyroid. Natural progesterone balances the thyroid inhibiting effect of estrogen dominance. Supplementation with thyroid glandular extracts, l-tyrosine, the Auyervedic herb, gulgulipid, licorice, maca and coleus forskolin are also effective.

Iodine is the major mineral that is essential for a healthy thyroid. It can either be taken as a supplement or obtained from iodine rich foods like seaweed and fish. In fact, eating seaweed on a daily basis is the best source not only of iodine but other essential trace minerals.

Dietary recommendations to support thyroid function include getting adequate protein i.e. organic beef, poultry, eggs, fish, and cultured milk products such as kefir and yogurt.

Thyroid healing foods are high in B vitamins such as wheat germ, whole grains, nuts, seeds, dark greens, legumes and Brewer's yeast. Include foods rich in selenium like fresh tuna, brazil nuts and the zinc-rich foods, pumpkin seeds, sunflower seeds and fish. Another great thyroid promoting food is coconut oil.

Unfortunately, the standard thyroid blood test often fails to pinpoint an underactive thyroid. Saliva testing for thyroid function provides a much more accurate picture.

There are also effective self-diagnosis tests. Using a basal thermometer, take an underarm temperature reading the in the morning before getting out of bed and moving around for five consecutive days. Leave it under the arm for 10 minutes. A low functioning thyroid will show an average temperature of under 97.5 F. However, do not test around ovulation since body temperature rises up at that time. Also check the resting pulse.

Less than 85 beats per minute plus a low basal temperature may indicate hypothyroidism.

Exercise is also an important thyroid health strategy. Sustained aerobic exercise raises the body temperature allows proper binding to the hormone tissues.

The liver is the body's most important detoxification factory. The liver is responsible for over 500 vital functions! One of its most important jobs is protecting your body from the invasion of thousands of toxins. The liver processes every foreign chemical that finds its way into the body so it can be safely eliminated.

The liver also helps to digest and assimilate fats, vitamins and minerals, provides fuel for the body, metabolizes drugs and alcohol, stores extra blood, maintains electrolytes, regulates sex hormones and creates immune-building substances.

Every system in the body is affected by your liver's health. Health problems associated with compromised liver function tend to be nonspecific ailments and often baffle conventional doctors. They include low energy, hormonal imbalances, poor sleep, digestive problems, obscure aches and pains, chronic fatigue, mental lethargy, and feelings of anger, frustration or depression.

When it comes to hormonal balance, the liver has a most important job to do. It is responsible for the breakdown and elimination of estrogens from the body. This includes both natural estrogen made by the body and environmental estrogens. If the liver is overwhelmed with too many pollutants, drugs or a lack of B vitamins, it may be seriously hindered in accomplishing its work.

When the liver is functioning properly, it will be able to effectively metabolize estrogen into a safe or "good guy" estrogen metabolite. This metabolite is considered a "good guy" estrogen because it binds weakly to cell receptors and has an anti-inflammatory effect as well as inhibitory effect on breast cancer.

If, however, the liver is compromised in its functioning, it will metabolize estrogen into a powerful estrogen by product. These are known as the 'bad guy' estrogen. This much stronger 'bad guy' estrogen will then be reabsorbed back into the body.

In essence, a woman becomes exposed to the same estrogen twice. The second time around it is a more potent form.

If there is a higher ratio of the 'bad guy' estrogen to the 'good guy' estrogen, the estrogen dominant condition will occur in the body with all the accompanying risks.

Researchers evaluated the effects of the 'bad guy' estrogen, on estrogen-sensitive breast cancer cells. They found when cultures of the breast cancer cells were experimentally exposed to the bad metabolite, they had the maximum stimulatory effect on DNA synthesis in the cells. The effect was nearly twice as strong as that induced by estradiol, the most potent of the body's three major forms of estrogen.

It was also discovered this bad metabolite strongly influenced the activity of special proteins that regulating the cell growth cycle. This causes the breast cancer cells to increase and divide much faster.

The 'bad guy' estrogen also promotes the transformation of the human papilloma virus, the precursor for cervical cancer, into the malignant type.[9]

High levels of the 'bad guy' estrogen have been linked to alcohol consumption, a sedentary lifestyle, a high-carbohydrate, high-fat diet, and increased body mass.

On the other hand, vigorous exercise, a healthy thyroid, hormone balance, and consumption of cruciferous vegetables encourage the production of the 'good guy' estrogen.

There is a class of plant chemicals called indoles which are helpful in promoting the conversion of estrogen into the safe metabolite and inactivate the toxic one. This is crucial protection from breast cancer and all estrogen dominant conditions. The indoles are found in cabbage, broccoli, brussels sprouts, kale, cauliflower, bok choy, kohlrabi, mustard and turnips. Flax seeds, omega-3 oils, onions and garlic also significantly increase the proper estrogen ratio. These foods should be eaten abundantly to support a healthy hormonal balance.

Indoles are also available as supplements either called I3C (indole-3-carbinole) or DIM(diindolylmethane).

Your body and brain are built of protein, water, fat, minerals and vitamins. Body parts (muscles, bones, nerves, bones) can be made only from water and solid foods like protein, minerals and fat. Without them, your body doesn't have the building blocks to replenish itself and replace worn out cells.

Carbohydrates have a very different function. They are the fuel your body uses. Yes, they're important, you cannot make muscle, hormones or bones out of carbohydrates.

Your body needs high quality carbohydrates to provide fuel for energy. Unfortunately, popular foods like bagels, pasta, donuts, candy bars, cakes and cookies are poor quality carbohydrates.

So what happens to all the sweets and starches you eat? They turn into blood sugar (glucose) while still in your mouth, shocking and alarming your whole system, "Get rid of it, fast!" shrieks your body. Out rushes insulin, made by your pancreas, from whatever protein you are eating. Insulin knocks every bit of the glucose high out of your bloodstream and quickly stores it as fat, where it gathers in you body, crowding your muscles and clogging your arteries

As you gain excess fatty weight around your middle from consuming too many carbohydrates, insulin gets less effective. The more carbs you eat, the more fat you store in your abdomen and the more insulin you need. Meanwhile your pancreas is running out of protein to meet the escalating demand for insulin because you aren't eating enough protein. You're filling up on carbs and sweets instead. Often, the end result of all this is diabetes or breast cancer.

Women with high insulin levels have a breast cancer risk almost three times higher than women with normal levels. Too much insulin can stimulate the growth of an already existing breast cancer. Insulin levels are often higher in women who are overweight, particularly if they carry weight around their waists. Contributing factors to high insulin include over consumption of sugar, alcohol, refined carbohydrates, and lack of exercise.

Insulin is released from the pancreas to reduce high levels of glucose in the blood. Its job is to bring down these levels and helps the glucose get into your cells where it can be used for energy. Fat cells make estrogen. The more weight one has, the more estrogen is made resulting in estrogen dominance.

Insulin interferes with the body's ability to properly convert hormones along their appropriate pathway. In some women this leads to an increase of male hormones, androgens, leading to Polycystic Ovarian Syndrome which causes acne, facial hair, irregular periods and infertility. It can also cause an excess of estrogen production, once again creating an estrogen dominant condition.

An interaction between estrogen and insulin may encourage the growth and proliferation of breast cancer cells. When breast cancer cells are chronically bathed with estrogen, the breast cancer cells are more susceptible and more sensitive to insulin, which stimulates the proliferative response of the cells.

A diet of high sugar, which results in excessive insulin production, is a time bomb to our health. It is especially dangerous to the health of children. The vicious cycle of a high sugar-high insulin syndrome in young children and teenagers goes like this. Overeating junk food makes you fat. Increased body fat and lack of exercise lead to high insulin levels. High insulin levels leads to further craving of sugary carbohydrates to generate energy for the body. More insulin is released in response to increased carbohydrate intake, leading to more weight gain. More body fat leads to more estrogens, which, in turn, lead to earlier breast development and menstruation.

The following are some helpful dietary guidelines.

Increase complex carbohydrates in your diet i.e., whole grains, vegetables, fruits, beans, seeds and nuts.

Have meals three times a day with healthy snacks in-between. Never skip a meal.

Make sure each meal includes some protein, healthy fats (olive oil, coconut oil, butter, flax seed oil) along with the complex carbohydrates.

Reduce the consumption of white flour products, sugar, sodas (including diet sodas), potatoes especially french fries and potato chips), artificial sweeteners and candy.

There is no longer any doubt estrogen dominance is an unrecognized risk factor for breast cancer. While estrogen dominance may have many causes, it will always create some degree of imbalance or discomfort. It shows up as a variety of hormonal problems, most often as the following conditions: PMS, endometriosis, polycystic ovaries, fibrocystic breasts, ovarian cysts, infertility and fibroids. Stressful situations, either physical or emotional, also contribute to an estrogen-dominant condition.

The degree of discomfort from these symptoms may vary. All of these conditions are indicators the body is seriously out of balance. Persistent and ongoing PMS is not a normal occurrence. Menstruation was never designed by nature to be a painful experience and PMS is certainly not an inherent liability of being a woman. These problems should neither be ignored nor medicated with pharmaceutical drugs. A healthy woman will not get PMS.

The seeds of dysfunction are sown early in a girl's life and they put young women at a greater risk of all types of chronic degenerative illnesses later in life. Without attending to the real cause, a woman may continue to experience ongoing physical and psychological problems that could, possibly, lead to more chronic hormonal imbalances, infertility, miscarriage, or the other health issues previously discussed.

It is a myth to believe by prescribing dangerous drugs such as the pill, Lupron or Prozac will help young women. In fact, prescribing drugs to suppress symptoms will ultimately make things worse or contribute to further health problems.

With so many challenges to maintaining healthy hormones, it's no surprise 90 percent of women experience PMS at some time in their lives. For some, the symptoms may be mild, for others they can be quite disturbing and distressing. PMS generally occurs in the last week or two before menstruation begins. This part of the cycle, known as the luteal phase, should be the time when progesterone levels are the highest. However, if a woman is experiencing stress, poor eating habits, a junk food diet, a toxic body or illness, the delicate reproductive system can be altered, giving rise to an imbalance; low progesterone and high estrogen levels.[1,2,3]

A study by Swedish researchers revealed the severity of PMS symptoms correlates with levels of estradiol during the luteal phase of the menstrual cycle. In addition to an increase in negative mood symptoms, higher luteal-phase estradiol levels were associated with increased headaches, swelling, and breast tenderness.[4] This study is one of the first to specifically link emotional and physical PMS symptoms with estradiol activity over the course of the entire menstrual cycle.

Other problems, such as endometriosis, are putting women at risk. Endometriosis, is a disease affecting as many as 10 million U.S. women in their reproductive years. Endometriosis occurs when tissue similar to the endometrium, the uterine lining, is also found in areas outside the uterus, such as on the lining of the abdomen and pelvis, the bowel, bladder and ovaries. The presence of this tissue can cause internal bleeding, scar tissue formation, inflammation, and can result in pelvic pain, painful menstruation, infertility, and abnormal vaginal bleeding. According to the results of an Endometriosis Association survey of 4,000 of its members, endometriosis sufferers appear to have an increased risk of breast cancer, melanoma, and ovarian cancer compared with other women.

Another common problem is Fibrocystic Breast Disease (FBD), which really could be called a condition of congestion, toxicity and excess estrogen build-up. This is usually due to poor blood and lymph circulation and an overload of the body's normal detoxification systems. It is a non-cancerous condition characterized by painful lumps or cysts. The pain can increase before menstruation. It is estimated that 50-80 percent of North

American women are affected. Some of the causes of FBD include estrogen dominance, poor blood and lymph circulation, toxic accumulation, underactive thyroid gland, nutritional deficiencies, poor digestion and assimilation, aggravating foods such as coffee, sugar and dairy, and emotional and physical stress. There is a saying in Oriental Medicine a Chinese doctor would rather see 10 men than 1 woman. Why? Because women's bodies are much more complicated. It is, therefore, imperative to use holistic modalities to address the underlying health issues. The following modalities are extremely beneficial: Traditional Chinese Medicine, Western and Eastern herbal medicine, clinical nutrition, homeopathy, naturopathy, chiropractic, aromatherapy, and osteopathy. Some form of stress management, meditation, exercise and emotional healing have also been extremely beneficial. As with all health problems, healing is really a holistic journey and requires change in diet, attitude, lifestyle, and detoxification. Whenever and wherever dysfunction is occurring in the body, the real need is to heal the underlying problems. Unfortunately, traditional medical doctors are ill-equipped and ill-trained to do this. It is extremely important to seek out the assistance of a competent and qualified holistic health practitioner to create a protocol for healing the body.

Practical tips to balance low progesterone/ high estrogen conditions:

1. Eliminate hormone-laden meats, non-organic vegetables, and fruits produced with pesticides
2. Daily eat indole-containing foods from the cruciferous family, broccali, brussel sprouts, kale
3. Eliminate all pasterized dairy products, coffee, sodas, black tea
4. Reduce sugar and high carbohydrate foods
5. Decrease alcohol, and transfatty acids, i.e. margarine and fried food
6. Increase fiber with seeds and nuts
7. Drink filtered water daily
8. Eat lots of fresh fruits and vegetables, healthy fats (olive oil, butter, flax seeds, coconut oil) and good quality proteins (fish, eggs, chicken, turkey, beef, lamb)
9. Use natural progesterone cream twice daily from day 15-25 of the menstrual cycle
10. Use liver supporting nutrients and herbs like milk thistle, artichoke, and dandelion
11. Use hormone-balancing nutrients like maca,chasteberry, black cohosh, Indole-3-carbi nol, DIM (diindolylmethane) flax lignans
12. Get at least 20-30 minutes of regular moderate exercise
13. Use stress relaxation or meditation in your daily routine

Traditional Chinese medicine has had more than two thousand years of success in treating cancer, and at least five hundred years effectively healing breast cancer. Its ancient understanding of the root causes underlying breast cancer is as valid today as it was in the past.

Chinese medicine is one of the most holistic medical systems presently available. One of its most enlightened aspects is it unites mind and body. To a practitioner, emotional or mental events are pieces of important diagnostic information to be gathered to help assess the patient. One of the most important principles of Chinese medicine is the understanding person and their symptoms are part of a whole pattern. Honora Lee Wolfe, Chinese practitioner and author explains how a practitioner views a patient.

> "She is like a landscape painting with various aspects – water, trees, mountains, etc.– but all of one piece. The practitioner then prescribes singularly or with a combination, acupuncture, herbal, nutritional, exercise and massage therapies to work effectively with the entire pattern. Done skillfully, Chinese medicine cannot separate a person into segmented parts treating one symptom or one part at the expense of the other. Each part is only relevant in relationship to the whole of each patient's personal 'landscape'."[1]

Any change, even one sign or symptom may change the entire pattern and, therefore, the entire treatment plan. In this way, Traditional Chinese Medicine is indeed a holistic and humane system of medicine.

One of the greatest strengths of Chinese medicine is its preventative approach. In this way, imbalances can be addressed long before they manifest as full-blown symptoms or diseases.

Western medicine doesn't really have a frame of reference to understand these subtle changes and generally chooses to ignore them. This is especially important in the treatment of gynecological disorders.

Western medicine, has no comprehensive model for the cause of breast cancer, offers no effective prevention nor has developed any safe, painless treatment for healing. Chinese medicine has developed a profound and comprehensive understanding and treatment protocol. From the Western perspective, breast cancer is a total mystery. From the Chinese medicine perspective there are clear, observable signs and symptoms that can be non-invasively treated. Breast cancer is understood as a grouping of underlying imbalances progressing to greater and greater disharmony.

Minor symptoms will eventually turn into major problems if not properly addressed. First, let's understand some basic concepts of the way Traditional Chinese Medicines views the root causes of breast cancer. From a TCM perspective, breast cancer has very obvious and treatable early warning signs. Breast cancer, like any disease, begins first as a Qi (pronounced 'chee') or energy problem. When women complain of vague, intermittent discomforts, not detectable by scientific tests, they are really speaking in the language of Qi. Some of these "energy disturbances" may show up as occasional breast tenderness or periodic headaches. After some rest or an aspirin these symptoms may disappear.

Western culture has conditioned us to believe these are insignificant events. They are not. Any weakness or imbalance in the body's energy will begin to cause functional problems in the organs. Symptoms may appear as menstrual problems, PMS, breast tenderness, migraines, mood swings and more. If not treated at the source, these physical symptoms can worsen and may lead to a precancerous condition. This is the time masses or tumors can appear, or a woman may experience infertility or develop endometriosis. Sat Dharam Kaur, N.D., further explains the process by which breast cancer can arise.

First there is stagnation of energy in the liver. One of the functions of the liver in Oriental medicine is to circulate the body's energy, which is known as Qi, freely in all directions. This energy can be blocked by suppressed emotions — holding onto anger, anxiety, worry, a long period of depression or frustration, or grief. These emotions will interfere with the smooth flow of energy in the liver, causing a blockage. Other variables contributing to liver stagnation include lack of exercise, shallow breathing and excess consumption of unhealthy fats. Qi stagnation may manifest as irregular periods, premenstrual breast swelling and pain, breast cysts, irritability, fatigue and depression. Qi stagnation is also often linked to a deficiency of blood in the liver or kidney.

Second, there is a stagnation of blood in the liver. As liver energy does not circulate freely, the blood the liver holds becomes stagnant. Energy moves the blood. If the energy flow is disrupted, the blood flow is impaired.

There will be reduced circulation to the breast area. In medical terms, the blood coagulates more easily than it should, or has increased viscosity.[2] "Another contributing factor to breast disease is the accumulation of dampness or phlegm. Phlegm arises from Qi stagnation affecting the function of the spleen. The role of the spleen in Chinese medicine is to transform and transport food to regulate the body fluids. The disturbance of the liver will affect the spleen so it is unable to perform this task effectively. A build-up of fluids will occur, and over time can form a soft mass or lump.

Eventually, the combination of Qi stagnation and phlegm accumulation may cause the mass to become more firm. The presence of an actual toxin encourages the mass to become cancerous. The toxins may be internally or externally generated.

Toxins can include but are not limited to environmental chemicals, pesticide residues, encrusted fecal matter and excess estrogen. After a period of time the stagnant Qi turns into heat or 'fire' and becomes what is known as toxic heat. The heat injures the blood and yin and the mass hardens, leading to a cancerous tumor. A soft lump indicates an accumulation of phlegm, while a hard breast lump is indicative of blood stagnation or toxic heat.

Accordingly, cancer prevention in Chinese medicine consists of effective means to treat depression, anger, anxiety, grief or other emotional factors interfering with the circulation of energy; avoid substances increasing the production of phlegm (such as unhealthy fats, wheat, dairy and sweets); improving circulation so stagnation will be kept to a minimum and elimination of toxins.[6]

Chinese medicine is able to detect and treat minor and subtle shifts of energy. They may only be noticed by a person as a slight uncomfortableness or seemingly insignificant physical symptoms or emotional imbalance, poor sleeping patterns or indigestion. If these imbalances are not addressed, or are treated with prescription drugs, a minor condition may become progressively more chronic.

Road Signs And How To Read Them

Now that we have the theory explaining how imbalances in the body may develop into more serious hormonal imbalances and diseases, let's look at how they occur for woman. To best illustrate this point, we'll explore the life history of a patient named Helen. Helen isn't a real person, but rather a composite, drawn from the health histories from the many women I have consulted with over the years.

In this fictional account, Helen, at 27 years of age, has just been diagnosed with breast cancer. We will unravel the many conditions in Helen's past contributing to this development. The story starts at the beginning of Helen's life, at conception.

Helen's mom, Cindy, was determined to be a successful lawyer. She went to a very competitive law school, studied long hours and even held down a part-time job. Her hardworking years at school awarded her a position at a top law firm. Starting as a new lawyer right out of law school, Cindy was swamped with work. She worked long hours, skipped meals, smoked, and lived on black coffee.

She had been on the pill since starting college. She met her husband at the law firm, another hardworking and competitive lawyer. After four years, Cindy decided it was time to start her family. Three months after stopping the pill she found out she was pregnant. Being a dedicated lawyer, she stayed at work right up until her ninth month. During her pregnancy she had morning sickness, was constantly fatigued, often moody, and had fluid retention. She did the best she could to eat healthily, but continued to smoke.

Helen came along after a long labor of 36 hours. She emerged a beautiful, bouncing baby girl. She was breast-fed for three months. When her mom went back to work and Helen was put into day care. Her mom expressed breast milk for another two months. Helen was put on a milk formula. She began eating solid foods by six months. She loved milk, cheese, ice cream and French fries. Soon persistent ear infections ocurred, followed by many courses of antibiotics. She had regular bouts of diarrhea, colic and became a very 'fussy' baby.

By the time she reached six years old, she was a vivacious and intelligent child who loved school, was allergic to many foods and was a rather "picky" eater. She also developed quite a sweet tooth demanding candy, cookies and soda daily. Although Helen's earaches had now disappeared, she did suffer from frequent colds, coughs and flu. Usually the doctor prescribed antibiotics, cough medicine or a baby aspirin.

Sometimes Helen experienced constipation and also had a frequent skin rash. Aside from these little problems, Helen was considered a healthy child. During her teenage years Helen experienced discomfort with her menstrual cycle. Her period started when she was 11 years old. Painful cramps and heavy clotting were common. She would often have to take Tylenol for the pain. Helen was on a constant roller coaster of mood swings before her periods, and would find herself either sulking or fighting with her parents. Eventually she was prescribed the pill to help regulate her periods. Helen suffered from hay fever and relied on antihistamines to get through allergy season.

Like most teenagers, Helen was constantly watching her weight, often skipping meals or grabbing a bagel on the way out the door. Her favorite drink was diet soda.

Helen made it into a top university. The academic demands were great so, she let her hair down partied on the weekends. She often drank too much alcohol, waking up with a hangover on more than one occasion. Helen had stayed on the pill since it was prescribed five years ago. In using it as a contraceptive, it also stopped the cramps and heavy bleeding, which would return with a vengeance if she went off the pill. She was always tired and having to pump herself up with several cups of expresso coffee the first thing in the morning.

Her allergies had gotten worse. She was becoming allergic to more and more things. Her moods were yo-yoing all over the place. She especially noticed getting crazier right before her induced monthly period. Her monthly PMS symptoms, bloatedness, sore breasts, weight gain, headaches and sugar cravings made her dread getting her period.

After graduating, Helen found a lucrative, exciting job. She worked long hours and skipped meals. When she was finally able to grab a meal, it was usually from a fast-food restaurant. She loved her job and worked long hours. She was still constantly tired, had severe PMS, and lumpy painful breasts. She also struggled with candida. Occasionally, right before her period, a migraine would hit. On one of her regular visits to her gynaecologist, she was diagnosed with endometriosis. Several years later, during a breast exam, a small pre-cancerous lump was discovered.

Understanding the Journey

So, how did Helen's personal history contribute to the development of a pre-cancerous lump, known as ductal carcinoma in situ? Angelo Druda, a master Chinese herbalist specializing in gynecology, offers his insights in deciphering this process from the perspective of Traditional Chinese Medicine (TCM).

In our examination of the health destiny of Helen, we begin with her mother, Cindy. The child must always deal with the inherited limitations and liabilities of the mother. The most common deficiency of pregnancy is blood and yin deficiency. The blood is the lifestream of the body, which carries nutrients to all the organs and cells. The yin is the deeper life essence of the body. If these deficiencies are not addressed in pregnant women, there is a danger the fetus will not be sufficiently nourished. Such failure to nourish the fetus can result in the child being born with an insufficiency of its prenatal inherited energy, life force and strength. This predisposes one to health imbalances in the course of life.

Cindy lived an active and stressful life. She not only toxified her blood with toxic by-products of stress chemicals, but through diet, using coffee and tobacco regularly.

Her past use of the pill may have also contributed to blood toxicity and to a pattern of deficiency in pregnancy. So, Cindy looks like the type of person who might have entered her pregnancy with a predisposition to blood and yin deficiency.

Even so, Helen seemed quite healthy and well at birth. Her early life history may not have been sufficiently nurturing, due to her premature separation from her mother at three months of age. There is no doubt the poor dietary practices directly contributed to her chronic ear problems. An infant has an undeveloped digestive system that needs to be properly nurtured and grown for health and longevity. Her diet was full of indigestible bovine fats, fried oils, and processed sugars. Such foods only increased her internal inflammation and her stomach's production of mucus and phlegm. Lying on her back for a good deal of the time, it was easy for this phlegm and inflammation to settle in the child's' middle ear.

This phlegmy condition should have been corrected with proper foods, such as whole grains and steamed veggies to warm the digestive fire and dry the dampness. All sugars should have been eliminated. A TCM pediatric formula could have been used to treat the infection and correct the digestive fire. Instead antibiotics were employed. The cold energetics of the antibiotics eliminated the bacteria, but only weakened her digestive fire and established a chronic tendency towards ear infections, colds and flu. Over time the weakened digestive system showed itself in regular bouts of diarrhea, colic, behavioral discomfort and allergies.

As Helen grew older, she followed in her mother's footsteps. Her persistently poor dietary habits continued to weaken her digestive system and toxify her liver. Her stress inhibited proper liver function. Using antibiotics for the colds and flu weakened her natural immunity over time, and exacerbated the digestive weakness and phlegm. She began to exhibit inflammation and heat in the large intestine, setting the stage for candida problems. With the onset of her first period at the age of eleven, the disharmony established in her early life began to exhibit itself in new and uncomfortable ways. Her toxic and stressed-out liver was now unable to relax and smoothly conduct the increased levels of bodily energy during her menstrual cycle. The energy tended to become stuck in the liver, creating mood swings and sometimes sore breasts. Rather than flowing smoothly through the body, the Qi or life energy, was now beginning to become stagnated in the breast tissue. Because she tended toward weak digestion and poor diet, her body had difficulty producing sufficient quantity of blood to serve the reproductive cycle. The stagnant liver energy compromised her blood circulation causing her pain during her period. The toxic nature of the blood caused it to stagnate and begin to thicken. The blood clots only exacerbated her menstrual pain.

It was in her youth Helen should have made the adjustments critical to her health. She should have changed her dietary and lifestyle habits to ensure proper liver and digestive function. Her menstrual cycle was a clear indicator something was very wrong but she ignored those signs and then doubted her ability to make those changes.

Finally she opted to use the pill to change her bodily pattern rather than addressing the root cause of the imbalance. The pill granted her some short-term symptomatic relief, but over time, it increased her tendency towards energy and blood stagnation and deficiency. This pattern could have been changed while she was young by modifying her diet, the judicious use of exercise and relaxation, and by choosing one of the many highly effective TCM formulas to harmonize the liver, stomach and spleen.

Because the pattern was not addressed, it gradually progressed from an energetic imbalance to actual organ dysfunction. Over time energetic imbalances will finally damage the soft tissue, the mucous membranes and even the genetic programming of our bodies. At this stage, healing becomes much more difficult. Helen's mood swings, allergies, bloatedness, headaches, weight gain, and sugar craving are dramatic signs of her body's call for help. The stagnation of blood and Qi has now led to neoplasms, endometriosis and finally the lump in her breasts. Her body is hurt and its healing will now be a challenge.

Fortunately Chinese medicine's long history in treating gynecological problems and breast cancer successfully will be able to assist Helen in dissolving the lump and also, more importantly, addressing the chronic underlying pattern of disharmony. If Helen chooses to follow the program designed by her practitioner for her unique set of symptoms, she will be able to establish greater physical and emotional harmony."

Every stage of disharmony can be attended to. The more chronic and debilitating the symptoms, the more out of balance the body has become and the longer it takes to re-establish harmony. Fortunately, the body has the ability to heal. The goal of Chinese medicine is to restore the whole person to equilibrium — physically, emotionally, mentally, and spiritually. The nature of holistic healing modalities such as Traditional Chinese Medicine, Ayurveda, homeopathy, naturopathy, herbalism, and chiropractic is to support the body to regain balance and harmony. Symptoms are viewed as inner messages from the body and the mind, revealing some part of a person's life is out of balance. By knowing how to read these symptoms and following the appropriate lifestyle changes, dietary regimes and holistic treatments, harmony can once again be established. All these modalities teach how to maintain balance on the tightrope of life.

If a teenager was experiencing hormonal problems, or if there is a history of breast cancer, it would be prudent to measure hormone levels, estrogen metabolism, breast health and the acid/alkaline state of the body. Even if there are no obvious symptoms of chronic disease, things may be brewing below the surface that may, eventually, spin your health out of control. Not having any observable or obvious symptoms does not necessarily mean you have an optimally functioning body. An ounce of prevention is always worth more than a pound of cure.

The following simple, inexpensive diagnostic tests are the most reliable ways to provide you with the information to assess the health and balance of your inner terrain. They are able to provide a picture of just how well your body is doing.

Keeping tabs on your health by establishing a baseline for females of all ages and an annual follow up will help monitor your health. Remember, chronic illness doesn't just happen. For a problem to occur, compromised functioning must have been brewing over a long period of time. These tests will allow you to more clearly assess the actual state of your health; then the most effective steps can be taken to correct the problem before serious health issues manifest.

Saliva Testing

Before you can correct a hormonal imbalance, you need to know which hormones are out of balance.

Two pounds of frothy stuff, known as saliva, flows through your mouth every day. It lubricates your throat and helps you swallow. It contains enzymes that break down carbohydrates and anti-bacterial agents to help fight infection.

Saliva is also fast becoming the diagnostic procedure of choice for measuring levels of steroid hormones in the body. This is an accurate test to monitor the steroid hormones progesterone, estradiol, testosterone, cortisol, thyroid, DHEA and melatonin.

Most likely your conventional medical doctor has either never heard of saliva testing or doesn't believe in its accuracy. Fortunately, the *World Health Organization* disagrees since it considers saliva testing to be the gold standard for accurately measuring hormones. Since 1983, more than 2500 papers and research articles dealing with salivary diagnostic tests have been published.

The test most doctors will prescribe to test hormones will

be a blood serum test. Blood tests are looking at compounds as they travel through the blood serum, most of which are protein-bound and not a reliable measure of accurate levels existing in the tissues.

In fact, blood tests are only able to measure a very small percentage, only 1- 9 percent, of the biologically active hormones circulating throughout the body.

Obviously, making a diagnosis based on erroneous results can be very dangerous. Unlike blood serum testing, saliva analysis is looking at the biologically active compounds, and saliva is truly representative of what is clinically relevant — the hormone levels in the cells. Health practitioners are able to predict, diagnose and correct many health problemsusing saliva testing.

Small molecules freely travel through the cells and into saliva ducts. It is these small molecules of various steroid hormones that are measured in saliva. Hormones present in the saliva reflect not only the biologically available hormones but much is entering tissues throughout the body. Saliva testing is the most accurate method of diagnosing hormone levels in the body.

Saliva testing provide a baseline for future reference and a diagnostic tool to investigate various health concerns. You can request your health practitioner to order these tests. Many saliva-testing laboratories do not require a prescription and up to six hormones can be ordered without a physician's reference. However, in order to properly interpret the results and devise a hormone balancing program, it is important to work with a qualified health professional.

Saliva collection is easy, non-invasive and collected at home. It merely requires spitting into a small tube, which then gets sent to a lab.

Monitoring Estrogen Metabolism

The Estrogen Metabolism Test, which uses a urine sample, is another home diagnostic tool able to identify estrogen-excess conditions. The following is a simplified explanation of what this test is measuring.

An important function of the liver is to metabolize estrogen so it can exit the body.

Depending on nutritional levels, toxicity, and liver function, the liver can metabolize estrogen into a benign "good guy" metabolite called 2alpha-hydroxyestrone (2-OHE1). This metabolite has anti-inflammatory effects and may even inhibit cancer growth. On the other hand, the liver can also metabolize estrogen into a more toxic "bad guy" form, called 16alpha-hydroxyestrone (16alpha-OE1), which can get reabsorbed into the body and potentially promote tumor growth. Elevated levels of 16alpha-OE1 are often found in women with breast cancer.

This diagnostic test shows how well the liver is metabolizing these two estrogen metabolites, as well as the ratio of the "good guys" to the "bad guys". If the ratio is in favor of the more toxic 16alpha-hydroxyestrone, then this is an important warning sign of increased risk for estrogen dominant conditions including hormone-dependent cancers.

The 2/16alpha-hydroxyestrogen ratios can also be modified through nutritional interventions including diet and supplementation. Cruciferous vegetables, i.e. broccoli, cabbage, cauliflower, mustard greens, brussels sprouts etc., protect against the "bad guy" estrogen. Supplements containing an active ingredient in cruciferous vegetables called indole-3-carbinole (I-3-C) or its metabolite Diindolymethnae (DIM) are equally protective. Ground flaxseeds also favorably benefit the 2/16 ratios along with adequate levels of B-Complex.

Women taking oral contraceptives or other types of

hormones would benefit from taking this test to monitor their estrogen metabolism. It is also recommended for women who feel they are at greater risk of developing breast cancer. This is an effective, inexpensive test and a preventive indicator of how well the body is clearing out the "bad guy" estrogens. If more of the toxic estrogen is circulating in the body, the more likely a woman may be confronting several estrogen-dominant problems such as fibroids, polycystic ovaries, endometriosis, and PMS etc. This test can only be ordered through your health practitioner.

It's All About Your Acid/Alkaline Balance

What if there was an inexpensive, effective and accurate home test that would allow you to daily monitor your risk of bone loss, gum disease, hormonal imbalance, inflammation, heart disease, cancer and your overall health status? Does that sound too good to be true? Well, in fact, there is a very simple way to keep tabs on your health. It's time to learn more about acid/alkaline testing!

But first, some basic understanding about acid/alkaline balance, also known as pH. In its natural healthy state, the body is slightly alkaline. It must maintain a slightly alkaline state for your very survival. The body has developed a complex system to keep it in balance.

Natural alkaline is produced by our boides until around thirty years of age. By the time we reach our forties, the majority of us have become overly acidic. Nearly everything we are exposed to (foods, environmental toxins, stress) produces acid and over time our buffer systems become less efficient at neutralizing that acid.

Unfortunately, in our modern world, a junk food diet heavily laden with acid-producing foods like sugar, soda and refined carbohydrates means even children are demonstrating high acidic levels.

The majority of fruits and vegetables leave an alkalizing effect. Think of apples, pears, and apricots, peaches, lemons, tomatoes, broccoli, cucumbers, squash beans, avocados, carrots, celery etc. Most grains and high protein foods are somewhat acid forming. Refined sugar is acid forming, while natural sea salt is alkaline-forming. Generally our diet should be composed of about 35 percent acid-forming foods and 65 percent alkali-forming foods.

Maintaining an alkaline balance is absolutely essential for good health. Individuals with a healthy acid/alkaline balance have physical vitality and stamina, mental clarity, a positive outlook, and resistance to and quick recovery from illness.

In contrast, overly acidic people are susceptible to numerous ailments, including fatigue, headaches, digestive problems, urinary tract conditions, chronic illnesses, colds and flu. A consistently acidic condition will predispose people to loss of minerals stored in the bones. Bacteria, fungus and parasites thrive in an acidic condition. An overly acidic condition reduces the amount of oxygen taken up by the cells. When a cell is oxygen deprived all sorts of serious health problems can be created including cancer.

An underlying metabolic acidity is a common denominator, and contributing factor to all degenerative and autoimmune diseases. An acid condition has several adverse effects on cell metabolism including impaired energy production, fluid accumulation, and an increase in free radical production.

Many organs and systems, especially the kidneys, adrenals and lungs, play important roles in maintaining proper acid/alkaline balance. Diet, however, is especially important. On a balanced wholefoods diet, the acid/alkaline balance is able to be maintained in proper proportion.

If you are overly acidic, you can bring your body chemistry into a healthier alkaline balance. It may take anywhere from six to twelve months to arrive at a consistent alkaline state. Heaping lots of vegetables on your plate and snacking on fresh fruit pumps up those alkalizing minerals. Cutting back on mineral-robbing candy, cakes, caffeine, sodas, ice cream and refined carbs reduces an acidic condition.

If you discover you are consistently acidic, it is suggested you consult with a complementary health practitioner to assess what might be compromising your metabolic functioning.

There is a very simple, inexpensive test able to measure your acid/alkaline levels on a daily basis, using paper pH strips. By checking the pH of your first morning urine, you will get an insight into your overall pH balance. When the first morning urine is between 6.5 (slightly acidic) and 7.5 (slightly alkaline), it indicates the overall cellular pH is appropriately alkaline.

Thermography – Seeing Into The Future

The most wisely promoted screening detection for breast cancer is mammography. However, this technology is not without its dangers, primarily, the cumulative exposure to DNA-damaging radiation. Mammography is not a particularly effective or safe diagnostic tool. Its shortcomings include the tendency for false readings and its inability to reveal unfavorable conditions when a breast lump is not present.

Fortunately, there is another option. It is called Digital Infrared Thermography (DIT) and is painless, non-toxic and highly accurate. It can safely be used to screen young women. Although you may have never heard of it, it has actually been used for over 30 years. In fact, over 80 peer-reviewed studies have proven its effectiveness. It is also FDA-approved for the use in breast cancer screening.

DIT requires neither radiation nor breast compression. As a diagnostic tool, it has the ability to detect breast irregularities and possible 'hot spots" years before they would ever be revealed with mammography or breast exam.

Thermography uses ultra-sensitive, high-resolution digital infrared technology. It is able to measure subtle changes in the temperature at the surface of the body. When a cancer is forming it develops its own blood supply in order to feed its accelerated growth. Since cancerous tumors have this increased blood supply, they are slightly hotter than the surrounding area in which they are found. The increased blood supply causes an abnormal heat pattern in the breast.

Thermography can detect this abnormal heat pattern by scanning the breasts with a specialized infrared camera. The information is then analyzed using sophisticated computer programs, which translate the data into anatomical images under the guidance of properly trained health professionals.

The difference in body temperature is measurable, particularly when both breasts can be compared. These abnormal heat patterns are among the earliest known signs of a potential cancer or inflammation. Any areas indicating increased heat can then be investigated further with a mammogram.

Thermography measures physiology, unlike a mammogram, which detects changes in anatomy. Often the physiological changes precede the anatomical changes. An unprecedented level of early detection can be realized when thermography is added to a woman's regular breast health care. It has been found an abnormal thermographic image is the single most important sign of high risk for developing breast cancer, eight times more significant than a first order family history of the disease. Studies show DIT has the ability to warn a woman of a developing cancer up to ten years before any other test.

A tumor must grow to about the size of a small grape before it will block enough x-rays to create an image on the film. DIT is the only screening method available that detects angiogenesis (the process whereby a group of blood vessels are specifically formed by a tumor to supply it with nutrients and oxygen). Thermography has the ability to detect a tumor's growth when it's size may be no larger than the head of a pin. This gives breast thermography the ability to detect cancer at its earliest and most treatable stage. it's truly an early warning system for the future risk of breast cancer.

DIT especially benefits young women since the breast tissue is more susceptible to the damaging effect of radiation, Thermography offers a much safer and more effective, screening alternative. A positive infrared scan may indicate the presence of many different breast abnormalities such as mastitis, benign tumors, fibrocystic breast disease, cancer, and others. Just as unique as a fingerprint, each patient has a particular infrared map of her breasts. Any change in this infrared map in future imaging can indicate an early sign of an abnormality.

This technology has an important role in breast cancer prevention. Thermography has the added ability to observe the influence of hormones on the breasts. Research has determined the single greatest risk factor for the future development of breast cancer is lifetime exposure to estrogen. In which case, controlling the influence of estrogen on breast tissue would be the single greatest method of breast cancer prevention.

While thermography does not medically, or legally replace mammography, it is certainly a valuable diagnostic tool.

Thermography has a unique role in the monitoring of a woman's breast health, since it has the ability to detect a precancerous state of the breast, or signs of cancer at an extremely early stage. Although not as readily available as mammography, the awareness and access to DIT is growing.

Getting your hormones back on track is not as difficult as you may think. The following suggestions provide effective solutions for the most common hormonal issues facing the modern woman. Natural hormonal support, hormone balancing nutrition and harmonizing life style choices, are the keys to hormonal health.

#1 Increasing Progesterone Levels

Since so many of the hormonal health issues affecting women are due to the imbalance between low progesterone levels and excessive estrogen levels, bringing those hormones back into their appropriate relationship is essential for good health. The use of natural progesterone is an effective and safe way to re-establish this delicate balance.

Natural progesterone is the term used to describe the bio-identical hormone made by the body. It is synthesized in a laboratory from an extract of wild yam or soy. Natural progesterone is the exact molecular match to the progesterone made by the ovaries.

Progestins, on the other hand, are progesterone-like chemicals that do not exist in nature. *The National Institute of Environmental Health Sciences* and the *World Health Organization* have classfied progestin as a know human carcenogens.

Progestins interfere with the hormonal signaling that prevents eggs from being released from the ovaries. Use of this drug has also been shown to lower levels of estradiol.

Also, ovarian cysts, endometriosis, fibroids and polycystic ovarian syndrome indicate that progesterone production is low.

The most popular progesterone products are available as creams, oils, and sublinguals. The most effective way to use progesterone is as a transdermal cream. Progesterone applications may require two to three months of use before maximum benefits are experienced.

Since every woman's body is unique, it is important to find the dose that works best for you. Women experiencing severe symptoms may initially require using more cream. It is considered safe to experiment until you find the dose that is correct for your body. However, it is best to use the lowest effective dose.

PMS and Progesterone

PMS is by far the most common complaint made by young women. Symptoms can include bloating/water retention, weight gain, breast tenderness and lumpiness, headaches, cramps, fatigue, irritability, mood swings, and anxiety. In women with severe PMS, irritability and mood swings can become outbursts of anger and rage. By definition, PMS symptoms usually occur in the two weeks before menstruation and sometimes, even, for a few days into menstruation.

While using natural progesterone can be quite effective in reducing or even eliminating PMS symptoms, it is by no means a magic bullet. Nothing is. However, since PMS is the result of poor nutrition, lack of proper sleep, lack of exercise, compromised digestion and immunity, physical and emotional stress, and environmental toxins, a holistic approach to healing is required. Each woman has her own unique response to hormonal imbalances. Some may be prone to migraines, others may feel tired and others may have irrational emotional outbursts. Whatever the symptoms, PMS is always an important sign of poor health and a unbalanced and harmful lifestyle.

How To Apply It

Natural progesterone is most readily absorbed when applied to the thinner-skinned areas of the body where the capillaries are plentiful. The best areas are the face, neck, chest, abdomen and the upper and inner areas of the arm and thigh. It can also be rubbed into the palms of the hands and the soles of the feet. Applying the cream at night can create a calming effect.

When To Use It

Application of natural progesterone follows the body's

natural progesterone production. Since menstruation is the time of the lowest progesterone levels, it is advised not to use at this time. In a typical menstruating woman, progesterone needs to be applied only from day 12 to day 26 of the cycle, using 15-20 mg per day applied twice a day, usually morning and night. Women who have a shorter or longer cycle than 28 days can find the appropriate day to begin using the cream by counting backward two weeks from the expected first day of the period and begin to use the cream at that time. This is because the length of time of the luteal phase, the last two weeks from ovulation to the beginning of menstruation, is almost always two weeks.

As the symptoms diminish, try reducing the amount of progesterone. If symptoms return, resume the previous dosage. Ultimately, the goal is to be hormonally balanced and symptom-free by incorporating dietary, nutritional and lifestyle strategies.

Other ways to help the body to increase its own progesterone production include supplementation with vitamin B6, vitamin E, boron, zinc, magnesium, selenium, the herb chaste tree berry and the Peruvian herb Maca. It is always advisable to monitor your hormone levels by using a saliva test.

#2 – Maca – The Miracle From Peru

Grown only in the high Andean plateau of Peru, Maca offers the Western world a truly miraculous plant. When grown and prepared organically, Maca is a vegetable so rich in minerals and nutrients which have a restorative effect on the endocrine system.

Maca is typically cultivated at approximately 14,000 feet above sea level and is the highest cultivated vegetable in the world. When farmed organically and prepared as a pre-cooked extract, Maca can be an extremely nutritious food. It contains substantial amounts of minerals such as calcium, magnesium, phosphorus, iron, zinc and the vitamin's B1, B2, B12, C, E and amino acid proteins.

According to Dr. Viana Muller, Ph.D., author of *Maca: Hormone Regulator for Women and Men — The Secret Royal Herb of the Incas* and herbal expert who first brought Maca to the American market, "Maca was originally called "ma" and was revered by women and used for hormone balancing during all the phases of a woman's life." Since that time, Maca has grown in popularity in the West. Researchers have found Maca promotes optimal functioning of the hypothalamus and the pituitary, thereby improving the functioning of all the endocrine glands.

Maca is effective by encouraging the ovaries and other glands to produce needed hormones. Unlike the phytoestrogenic herbs and foods, such as soy isoflavones, Maca does not contain any plant hormones. Through its plant sterols and lipids, it helps the glands make a better balance of its own hormones.

Maca has proven to be a very successful solution in assisting a variety of hormonal imbalances including irregular menstrual cycles, extremely painful periods, mood swings, PMS, fibroid tumors, endometriosis, headaches, depression, food cravings, excessive facial hair growth, missed periods and acne.

Native Peruvian women have traditionally used Maca to solve all types of female hormonal imbalances infertility and miscarriage. While there are many Maca products presently available on the market, most of them are farmed with chemical fertilizers and pesticides, powdered and then irradiated to prolong shelf life. This is the quickest and cheapest way to produce Maca. However, native people only grew it in the time-honored organic way.

Using organically grown Maca is critical because pesticides and irradiation can negate it's benefits. Maca is best used in an extract form. Recent research has confirmed an extract (cooked with boiling water) is more effective than the raw ground-up form generally found in most health food stores.

Maca has a malty and nutty flavor, and can be added to protein, fruit drinks, sprinkled on cereal or mixed with yogurt. It can also be added to warm water as a pleasant-tasting tea.

According to Dr. Muller, "Dosage is an important issue, not because of toxicity, but because it has powerful hormonal effects. In general, it is desirable to find the minimum effective dosage for the particular problem and to maintain this dosage for two or three months. In most cases, the initial dosage should be on the low side, either one or two capsules of 500 mg. or 1/3 tsp. of loose powder. The same low dosage should be maintained for the length of one cycle, in order to evaluate its effectiveness. If the problem is irregular or skipped periods, a higher dosage can be used. Below are some general guidelines for using Maca."

Irregular Menstrual Cycles

Young women who are experiencing irregular menstrual cycles need not go on birth control pills to regulate their periods. One to two teaspoons or six to twelve capsules of Maca root extract powder will usually bring on menstruation within two to four weeks.

Painful Menstrual Periods

One to two capsules (1/8 — 1/4 tsp.) a day for the entire month. Alternatively: 6-12 capsules (one to two tsp.)when the very painful menstrual cramps begin, when the period starts once or twice a day. Use this method sparingly only for as long as necessary.

Skin Eruptions – Acne

One to two capsules (1/8 — 1/3 tsp. powder) daily

PMS

One to two capsules (1/8 — 1/3 tsp. powder) daily. This will help relieve the "blues," bloating and headaches.

Ovarian Cysts

Two capsules (1/3 tsp. powder) daily until the cyst has dissolved. It might be necessary to use a higher dosage. Since ovarian pain can result from a number of different conditions and may not indicate a cyst, remember the importance of proper diagnosis and monitoring by a competent health care professional.

Endometriosis

Two capsules (1/3 tsp. of powder) daily help reduce pain and bleeding. However, the dosage can vary considerably.

#3 Extra Nutritional Support

Healthy hormones require a healthy diet. In addition to eating a wide variety of vegetables, fruits, good quality proteins, healthy fats and plenty of water, the following are some supplements that can help alleviate specific problems.

Vitamin E (400-1600 IU daily) helps alleviate PMS.

Chaste Tree (225-mg daily of a standardized extract) alleviates cramping and breast pain.

Essential Fatty Acids from either cold pressed flax seed oil (1-2 tsps) or ground flax seeds (2-3 tsp) or fish oil ((3-12 grams) help to reduce stress, inflammation and depression. It is also helpful for ovarian cysts and polycystic ovarian syndrome.

Magnesium (500-600 mg daily) Helps with PMS, moods and reduces inflammation. Magnesium needs to be used with calcium.

Calcium (1,000-1200 mg daily). Reduces moodiness, water retention, food cravings and pain.

Gamma Linolenic Acid or GLA (found in evening primrose oil) reduces breast tenderness, fluid retention, anxiety, bloating, headaches and mood swings.

Grape Seed Extract (50-200 mg daily) reduces swelling and fluid retention.

Cramp Bark (60 mg daily) alleviates menstral cramping prior to and during menstruation.

B-6, B-12 and the entire B-complex (50-100 mg) raises progesterone levels, balances moods, reduces PMS, improves fertility, relieves bloating and skin eruptions.

Liver cleansing nutrients, which help with proper estrogen metabolism — milk thistle, dandelion, choline, inositol, methionine. Indole-3-Carbinole (I3C), Diindolymethnae (DIM), and flax lignans.

#4 – Exercise

If you have a preteen or teenage daughter who is a junk food eating couch potato, it's essential to get her involved in some type of exercise whether it's team sports, roller blading, hiking or dance. In addition to the more physical forms of exercise, ancient forms of exercise and healing such as yoga and tai chi have a long and profound tradition of stretching and disciplining the body in ways that build strength, flexibility, emotional balance and inner peace.

Young children as well as teenagers can benefit from these practices. One of the most important reasons for encouraging young girls to exercise is to help delay puberty. Exercise has been shown to decrease the flow of estrogens and narrows the window of vulnerability to breast cancer. Clinical studies have shown young women who are involved in regular exercise and vigorous aerobic exercise programs begin puberty at an older age and have a nearly twofold decreased risk of developing breast cancer later in life.

A great way to tackle a moody girl is to get her body moving. There is hardly anything better for improving moods during the female hormonal cycle than exercise. In a recent study at Duke University, researchers found that three 30-minute workouts each week brought as much
relief as antidepressant drugs.

Michael Gurian, therapist, educator and best-selling author of the *Wonder of Girls* is emphatic about the need for girls to exercise. "For today's six-year-old who get lots of spontaneous running exercise, no other exercise may be necessary; by eight, however, an organized program (karate, soccer, swimming) would probably be beneficial; by twelve, perhaps more than one. At fourteen or fifteen, a girl will generally make her own decisions about participating in athletics. If she is developing physical issues, it is essential to try to encourage her to take up some kind of exercise."

Benefits of exercise:

> Lowers insulin levels
> Maintains balanced hormone levels, improves metabolismof estrogen
> Keeps cellular waste moving for elimination
> Increases metabolism and improves mood
> Helps curb cravings

Increases energy level
Enhances immune system
Increases bone density

#5 – Water of Life – Precious Water

When it comes to rebalancing the body, the most crucial ingredient is generally overlooked. That is the most precious, life-giving element on this planet, water! Did you know water is necessary for optimum brain function, digestion, and absorption of nutrients, circulation, hormonal management and all biochemical processes in each of your cells? It is also excellent for healthy, clear, soft skin.

Scientific research has shown the better water is managed in a cell, the more efficiently proteins, enzymes, hormones and other biochemical elements are able to function. Dehydration can create an imbalance of minerals, which will disrupts hormone balance.

Of particular and critical interest to women is the role of chronic dehydration in the development of breast cancer. In his book, *Your Body's Many Cries for Water*, Dr. Batman-chelidj says the stress created by dehydration "will increase the secretion of a hormone called prolactin which can cause the breast to transform into cancerous tissue. Dehydration alters the balance of amino acids and allows more DNA errors during cell division." Dr. Batmanchelidj goes on to say, "The breast is a water-secreting organ. Whether you are having a child or not makes no difference. The breast must be ready to fulfill its predestined role. If a woman already has breast cancer, drinking plenty of water would assist with any therapy by flushing out the toxins. If you do not have breast cancer or want to prevent a metastasis from occurring, it is urgent you drink enough water. If you don't, your breast may suffer horribly because of its unique role in supplying fluids."

A serious problem these days is a chronic state of

dehydration in women. When thirsty it is common to drink coffee, tea, fruit juices, sodas and energy drinks. Unfortunately this will contribute to dehydration. Only pure water will do!

#6 – Finding a Peaceful Heart

According to Chinese wisdom, the 'Heart is the King', overseeing the energy activity of your whole body: physical, emotional, mental and spiritual. The heart is the controlling message center for all your organs and has a profound effect on the whole realm of the body and mind.

If the King is upset, he will pass along his unhappiness to all the other organs. This is not merely a mental concept but, a physiological process understood for millennia.

A peaceful heart can help all the other organs function harmoniously. On the other hand, stress is the enemy of good health and a sense of well-being. Daily frustrations, pent-up emotions, rushing from one place to the next, working long hours, skipping meals, attending to an endless list of activities and demands, all contribute to high stress levels. Children and adults are succumbing to the demands of a frantic culture. Stress hormones are being pumped out continually, altering every single system of the body. If the body is out of balance, so are the emotions. The ability to respond calmly, optimistically and joyfully is jeopardized.

Constant stressful living and negative emotions also create another potential health problem. According to Chinese Medicine, stress and anger are the root cause of breast cancer. Making the heart peaceful may seem like an enormous task. Our modern, hectic lives seem to conspire against a peaceful heart. That is why every effort needs to be made to invite peacefulness into our heart.

Both adults and children would benefit from learning the importance and the techniques of nurturing a peaceful heart. There are many powerful and effective ways to foster more inner peace. It's just a matter of choosing the way that most suits your lifestyle and inclinations. These are not religious practices, but rather self-healing strategies. Such healing modalities encompass many ways including yoga, tai chi, Qigong, listening to relaxing music, walks in nature, swimming, contemplation, prayer or meditation.

Classes in many of these techniques are easily found in most neighborhoods. There are also many books, audio-tapes and videos that can instruct you in the privacy of your own home.

The goal is to settle one's thoughts, center within and apply the brakes to those stress hormones. Science is now acknowledging what the ancient healing traditions have known for thousands of years, the mind-body connection is a most potent healing force. It is important to remember that a little goes a long way.

Dr. Nan Lu, a classically trained doctor of traditional Chinese medicine and author of *Traditional Chinese Medicine — A Guide To Healing From Breast Cancer*, believes meditation is the best healing exercise. "Meditation is a superior way to reduce excess mental activity and repair yourself from the inside out. Meditation is something you can do any time, anywhere, and under any condition. There are walking mediations, sitting meditations, and standing meditations. Meditation is the one thing you can do for the rest of your life. It requires no special machine, place, time, or clothing. If you make meditation a regular part of your life, I believe you will see tremendous health benefits.

Breathing is another gateway to a peaceful heart.
Proper breathing is a vital key for reducing stress, creating balanced hormones, increased energy, and harmonious emotions. Proper breathing returns your body to balance. Filling your body with oxygen is filling it with Life Force. No wonder the conscious use of the breath has been an intrinsic part of all the ancient healing traditions throughout history.

The key to receiving the healing benefits from the breath is to breathe properly. Most people tend to breathe rapidly, shallowly and bring the breath only into their upper chest while raising their shoulders when they inhale. This is actually called futile breathing and turns out to be quite detrimental to good health. Dr. Saul Hendler, author of *The Oxygen Breakthrough — 30 Days To An Illness-Free Life*, states futile breathing can cause cardiac symptoms, angina, respiratory symptoms, gastro-intestinal distress, anxiety, panic, depression, headache, dizziness, seizures, increased susceptibility to infection and other immune dysfunctions, sleep disturbances, confused thinking and emotional upset.

To receive the maximum benefits from the power of the breath, you need to once again learn to a breathe properly! So, what exactly does that mean? To breath fully and deeply, requires drawing the breath all the way down into the bottom of the lungs, expanding the diaphragm. Imagine inflating the lungs as though you were filling up the bottom portion of a long balloon. The breath is drawn deeply into the belly. You know you are doing this correctly when you take a full, relaxed breath without lifting your shoulders!

Remembering to take several deep breaths whenever you encounter a stress event or thought, when you are in prayer or meditation, or while exercising, will have almost instantaneous results in restoring a peaceful heart. Finding and keeping a peaceful heart is truly one of life's greatest treasures.

Health is more than just the absence of illness. Health is the sum total of a body with all of its functions working in harmony. Symptoms tend to appear only after the body has been under duress for a period of time. Deprive the body of true sustenance long enough, and health problems are bound to occur. The goal is not just to repair health but, to build a strong, healthy body immune to illness. The fewer drugs children are exposed to, the healthier adults they will be.

Traditional medicine excels at suppressing symptoms, primarily with the help of pharmaceutical drugs. However, suppressing symptoms is not the same as restoring health. The risk comes from the toxic burden all drugs place on the body. All drugs have side-effects and some of the side-effects can be far worse than the condition for which they were initially prescribed.

While medical doctors are experts at suppressing symptoms, holistic health practitioners are trained in the paradigm of treating the whole person by restoring the body to balance. Symptoms disappear as the true needs of the body are properly identified and attended to. This is the definition of healing. Holistic medicine is also adept at treating all persons as the unique individuals they are. One size never fits all.

Competent and qualified holistic practitioners are our true healing allies on the journey to restoring health and balance. Their expertise incorporates such modalities as nutrition, acupuncture, herbs, homeopathic remedies, therapeutic massage and aromatherapy. Realigning the body with chiropractic and osteopathic adjustments supports the flow of healing energies.

As the interest and awareness in holistic medicine grows, there are many effective modalities to choose from. They include naturopathy, Traditional Chinese Medicine, Auyurveda, clinical nutrition, homeopathy, Western and Eastern herbal medicine, aromatherapy, chiropractic, osteopathy, mind-body healing and stress management techniques. Often a combination of therapies yields the greatest results.

In the old Wild West movies when a band of hostile enemies were set to attack the wagon train, the Wagon master would yell, "Circle the wagons! Circle the wagons!" The wagons would suddenly change their course and huddle into a protective circle providing protection and defense.

In a way, it's time for women to 'Circle the Wagons'. More than ever we live in a hostile world. It often appears we're surrounded and under unrelenting assault on all sides – from the polluted environment, toxic foods, media brainwashing, corporate interests and cultural demands. These forces seem in be incredibly daunting and inescapable.

Have we become the proverbial frog cooking in the pot. Are we floating so comfortably in the water our senses are dulled to the rising temperature? How long can we ignore the fact 80-90 percent of all cancers are due to environmental and food carcinogens? What do we say when it is now known that every child today is born tainted with foreign chemicals in their bodies? What are we to do when carcinogenic chemicals permeate breast milk, infuse our children's clothing, leach from their baby bottles, and are sprayed on their playgrounds? Why do we tolerate schools providing the poorest quality, most nutritionally depleted food to our children? How we can allow our teenage daughters to believe carcinogenic oral contraceptives are a better option than their own natural menstrual cycles?

Are we all blind to the fact that the health of all our children is in crisis as never before? Can we truly allow this state of affairs to continue?

Protecting the health of our children and guarding their hormonal well-being at every stage of their development is a profound responsibility. It is also a huge task, but not an impossible one. When it comes to making change happen, women have been unstoppable forces throughout history, whether within the family, within the community or within the world.

More than ever, now is the time for the voices of women to be heard.

The very first step must be the lifting of the veil of ignorance. We must question, challenge, investigate and trust our own inner knowingness. Making informed decisions is always dependent on a concerted effort to search for and uncover the truth. Becoming knowledgeable on matters relating to health, healing and the environment will allow you to be more discerning, sifting fact from fiction.

Once armed with this knowledge, the next step is to initiate the necessary changes to allow your children to be properly nourished and cared for on all levels.

At first, these changes may begin as small steps. Perhaps it's replacing all commercial, chemical household cleaners with safe, non-toxic ones, or eliminating all candy from the cupboard or adding organic vegetables to the meals. Every little bit of change helps, even if they are teeny, tiny baby steps of change. With each little bit, a stronger fabric of health is woven.

In Native American culture it was the wisdom and guidance of the grandmothers, the wise women elders, that looked after the welfare of the tribe far into the distant future. Their concerns and decisions were made with the future generations in mind. As nourishers of life, it is the nature of women to fiercely protect the well-being of children. The real life-sustaining values and concerns of women are far beyond the world of greed, politics and war.

The collective voices and wisdom of women are required to restore balance and to protect our daughters and sons from the consequences of a toxic world.

The voices were loud in Israel. In 1978, following a public outcry and threatened with legal action, Israel banned many toxic chemicals such as DDT and PCB's that were directly linked in a 1976 study with breast cancer in women. Once Israel banned these chemicals, they began noting a significant decrease in the level of toxic chemicals found in human breast milk. Over the next 10 years, the rate of breast cancer deaths declined sharply, with a 30 percent drop in mortality for women under 44 years old, and an 8 percent overall decline. Loud voices protesting the use of toxic chemicals polluting the water, food and air must pierce the silence. Defiant voices demanding food sources be pure, nutritious and in harmony with nature must become deafening. Strong voices that will not tolerate the poisoning of the unborn or the damaging of our children's bodies must be resolute in their determination.

There is much to be done. The lives of our children are precious beyond all words. With their long-term health and hormonal well-being presently in jeopardy, the time is well past due for all women to become the dynamic forces to make this world safe and healthy once again.

The strength and power of our collective voices must be heard. We are the voices that will restore sanity and balance to the world our children, our children's children and our great-grandchildren's children will inherit.

You are the powerful voice the children of the future are listening for.

Sherrill Sellman, N.D.

Sherrill is a naturopath, psycotherapist, health educator/ researcher and a passionate advocate for women's natural healthcare. For the past 27 years, she has traveled extensively throughout the world, sharing her knowledge, wisdom and practical solutions for the many health issues presently facing women of all ages.

She is a contributing editor/ writer for publications in Australia, New Zealand, Italy, Canada, United States, Germany, Netherlands and England. She is also a popular lecture and seminar presenter. Sherrill continues her global travels to alert women, work on her research and she rollerblades whenever possible!

For more information about Dr. Sellman's programs, lectures and tours or to inquire further into the topics explored in her books, visit http://www. ssellman.com or contact her at golight@earthlink.net.

Her free monthly newsletter is available by subscribing at http://www.ssellman.com

Women's Hormonal Health
Support Resources

Professional Health Practitioner Organizations

American Association of Oriental Medicine
866-455-7999 http://www.aaom.org

American Association of Naturopathic Physicians
866-538-2267 http://www.naturopathic.org

American College for the Advancement of Medicine
http://www.acam.org

American Institute of Homeopathy
888 445-9988 http://www.homeopathyusa.org

National Directory of Chiropractic
800 888-7914 http://www.chirodirectory.com

Children's Nutritional Supplements

Baby's Jarro-Dophilusa
This probiotic formula contains superior, scientifically documented probiotic strains and is an excellent probiotic formula for both newborns and infants. These products are available in health food stores or http://www.jarrow.com

BroccoMax
Cruciferous vegetables such as broccoli offer antioxidant and cellular protection. Broccoli seeds contain sulphoraphane, a powerful healing, anti-cancer ingredient which increases the activity of the liver enzyme responsible for deactivating or destroying carcinogens and removing them from your body. It also impedes the spread of tumors.

KIDS Multi
A chewable daily complete chewable daily complete vitamin and mineral supplement for children ages 2 to 12 . It contains no sugar.

Max DHA
The predominant fatty acid in the brain, nervous system and retina of humans is DHA, an omega-3 fatty acid. DHA is necessary for fetus and infantile neurological development during pregnancy and lactation.

Menstrual Health Nutritional Supplements

Jarrow Formulas
Manufacture a wide selection of excellent and innovative nutritional products. (available from health food stores or http://www.jarrow.com)

Flax Essence
A concentrated form of flax lignans that delivers ups to 30 times more lignans than other flaxseed products. Lingams are essential for restoring hormonal balance as well as helping the liver to properly metabolize estrogen into a safe, protective metabolite. http://www.jarrow.com

L-Theanine
This amino acid, a derivative of one of the brain's neuro- transmitters, is best known for creating a sense of relaxation by reducing stress and anxiety. It has shown to be an effective nutrient to successfully reduce the physical, mental and social effects of PMS. It also supports quality sleep.
http://www.jarrow.com

MenstraCalm
Combines natural phytonutrients, herbs, vitamins and minerals to provide support before and during monthly menstrual cycle.
http://www.jarrow.com

Women's Multi
Specially formulated to meet the nutritional requirements of women pre-imenopause. Its comprehensive formulation incorporates the latest research on vitamins, minerals and phytonutrients.
http://www.jarrow.com

Herbasway
Formulates a unique range of great tasting organic herbal and vitamin products as liquid tea concentrates.
http://www.herbasway.com or 800-672-7322

HormoneFactor
An herbal tea concentrate tht contains natural plant extracts from both the East and the West to combine the medicinal heritages of both traditions. A standardized herbal tea extract that helps to relieve cramps and discomforts associated with PMS. Also alleviates bloating, cramping, fatigue, mood swings and food cravings. It can be added as a great tasting tea to either hot or cold water. http://www.herbasway.com or 800-672-7322

Liver Enhancer
Liver Enhancer nurtures and detoxifies the liver, which helps to balance hormones, fights oxidizing free radicals and strengthens your immune system. http://www.herbasway.com or 800-672-7322

MultiVitamin Magic
A liquid concentrate of vitamins., which contains 100% daily values of the following vitamins: Vitamin A, Vitamin B1, Vitamin B2, Vitamin B3, Vitamin B5, Vitamin B6, Vitamin B12, Vitamin C, Vitamin D, Vitamin E, Vitamin K1, Niacin, Biotin, and Folic Acid. http://www.herbasway.com or 800-672-7322

HerbaGreen Tea
A great tasting caffeine-free green tea liquid concentrate, which is a powerful antioxidant, that helps maintain a strong immune system as well as protects against cancer, diabetes and weight gain.
www.herbasway.com or 800-672-7322

Vitamin Research Products
http://www.vrp.com or 800- 877-2447

HerBalance I
Relieves premenstrual symptoms such as fluid retention, breast tenderness, and loss of sex drive, depression, headaches and abnormal menstrual bleeding. Standardized extract of Vitex, Dong Quai, Alfalfa and blue cohosh work to normalize menstrual cycles.
http://www.vrp.com or 800- 877-2447

Organic Maca Products

Maca Magic
http://www.macamagic.com

WholeWorld Botanicals
888 757-6026 http://www.wholeworldbotanicals.com

Acid/Alkaline Testing

Swanson pH Balance
http://www.swansonvitamins.com

The Body Monitor
http://www.nancyappleton.com

Saliva Testing

Body Balance
828-285-226 http://www.bodybalance.com

Diagnos-techs, Inc.
800 878-3787 http://www.diagnostechs.com

Great Smokies Diagnostic Laboratory
800 522-4762 http://www.gsdl.com

ZRT Laboratory
503 466-2445 http://www.salivatest.com

Canada
Rocky Mountain Analytical Laboratory
Calgary, AB, Canada
866-370-5227 http://www.rmalab.com

Estrogen Metabolism Testing
Great Smokies Diagnostic Laboratory
(800) 522-4762 http://www.gsdl.com
Metametrix Clinical Laboratory
800.221.4640 http://www.metametrix.com

Thermography Resources

Breast Theromgraphy.Com
http://www.breastthermography.com
International Academy of Clinical Thermography
http://www.iact-org.org

Meditherm
http://www.meditherm.com

Natural (Bio-identical) Progesterone
Natural (bio-identical) creams are available over-the-counter only in the United States. In all other countries, it must be prescribed by a physician and then formulated by a compounding pharmacist. However, it usually can be ordered from the U.S. for personal use. The following companies provide excellent progesterone cream products.

Aarisse Health Care Products
Progestaplus 800 672-9329 http://www.healthyhormones.com

Optimal Natural Health
Bliss Cream 888-641-2547 http://www.optimalnaturalhealth.com

Organic Excellence
Organic Excellence Natural Progesterone Cream
http://www.organicexcellence.com

Natural Sweetener Alternatives

Stevia

The Stevia Plus brand, unlike other brands, contains no added malto-dextrin – an extremely high-glycemic substance. Instead it is enhanced with FOS, natural substances that nourish the growth of friendly bacteria. Stevia Plus is available as a powder, liquid or tabs. It is available in most health food stores. http://www.mothernature.com

Lo Han

HerbaSweet is an all natural sweetener which contains known for its prebiotic properties. This great tasting formula has nocalories and can be a natural addition to coffee, tea, cerealsand for baking and cooking. http://www.herbasway.com

Lo Han Sweet is a powder that combines Lo Han and xylitol. It is low on the glycemic index, heat stable and low in calorie. It can be used to sweeten drinks for cooking and baking. http://www.jarrow.com

Xylitol Products

Unique Sweet

All-natural xylitol crystals for one-to-one substitution with ordinary sugar. http://www.vrp.com

Xylitol Unique Gum and Mints

Chewing gum and mints come in a wide assortment of flavors made only with xylitol. http://www.vrp.com

Healthy Food

Eat Wild

The clearinghouse for information about pasture-based farming. Also provides sources for products throughout the U.S. http://www.eatwild.com

Rawmilk
Provides education and resources about organic, raw milk products
http://www.rawmilk.org

A Campaign for Real Milk
Provides education and resources about organic, raw milk products
http://www.realmilk.com

Teeccino Herbal Coffee
Herbal coffee is a great healthy substitution for coffee made with a blend
of herbs, nuts, fruits and grains that are roasted, ground and brewed just
like coffee. http://www.teeccino.com

Fertility Awareness and Menstrual Health Resources

Natural Fertility Websites

Ovu -Tech Fertility Detector
The Ovu-Tech is a hand-held mini-magnification lens about the size
and shape of a lipstick holder that is an easy way to monitor hormonal
changes and enhance menstrual cycle awareness.
http://www.beyondfertility.com

Natural Menstrual Aids
Diva International Menstrual Aid
http://www.divacup.com

The Keeper Menstrual Cup
http://www.keeper.com

Lunapads
http://www.lunapads.com

Toxic-Free Baby and Personal Care Products

Arbonne International
http://www.arbonne.com

Aubrey Organics
http://www.aubrey-organics.com

Burts Bees
http://www.burtsbees.com

JASON Natural Cosmetics
http://www.jason-natural.com

Neways International
http://www.neways.com

Women's Health Resources

Breast Cancer Action
Breast Cancer Action gives a voice to the women affected by breast cancer. It is the only national breast cancer organization that accepts no funding from the government or companies that profit from cancer.
877 278-6722 http://www.bcaction.org

National Women's Health Network
The National Women's Health Network improves the health of all women by developing and promoting a critical analysis of health issues in order to affect policy and support consumer decision-making.
202.628.7814 http://www.nwhn.org

Society for Menstrual Cycle Research

It is a source of guidance, expertise, and ethical considerations for researchers, practitioners, policy makers and funding resources interested in the menstrual cycle and pioneers the importance of menstrual cycle research to women's health.
http://www.pop.psu.edu/smcr

The Seventh Woman Foundation

The Seventh Woman Foundation's purpose is to disseminate information on women's hormonal issues. It has produced an excellent video series "Changing Your Life Through Understanding Your Hormones"
301 460-4222 http://www.theseventhwoman.org

The Young Survival Coalition

The Young Survival Coalition (YSC) is the only international, non-profit network of breast cancer survivors and supporters dedicated to the concerns and issues that are unique to young women and breast cancer.
http://www.youngsurvival.org

The Weston A. Price Foundation

The Foundation is dedicated to restoring nutrient-dense foods to the human diet through education, research and activism.
202.333.HEAL http://www.westonaprice.org

Women's Health Websites & E Newsletters/Digests

HormoneWise e-Digest

Dr. Sherrill Sellman's - HormoneWise e-Digest. A monthly newsletter, which provides articles, interviews, studies, and news stories offering a comprehensive overview of the many natural and effective approaches to women's hormonal health and well-being.
http://www.sssellman.com

Mercola Newsletter
One of the most comprehensive and educational newsletters available on holistic health solutions. http://www.mercola.com

Health Sciences Institute
Its mission is to keep you immediately informed of the newest and best in alternative medicine, so you can take control of your own health. http://www.hsibaltimore.com

Grassroots Environmental Education
A non-profit organization dedicated to researching and disseminating information about pesticides and other toxins and their impact on human health and the environment. They have produced a 30 minute documentary video (DVD) "Our Children at Risk" a which explores the latest scientific research linking environmental toxins to children's health problems. http://www.grassrootsinfo.org 516 883 0887

PCOS Health Review
Provides natural therapies and self-help strategies for ovarian cysts and polycystic ovarian syndrome. http://www.ovarian-cysts-pcos.com

Herbasway Health and Nutrition Journal
Updates from the latest scientific research about health related topics as well as tips for improving your lifestyle, health and well-being. http://www.herbasway.com

Thyroid Newsletter
A comprehensive website about all aspects of thyroid health, thyroid imbalances and effective solutions. http://www.thyroid.about.com

Total Health Magazine
Provides excellent articles on leading edge information regarding health and healthy solutions. http://www.totalhealthmagazine.com

Menstruation.com.au
Its aim is to provide information, products, and an alternative viewpoint about menstruation so that you can feel great about being a woman every day of the month! http://www.menstruation.com.au

Holy Hormones Honey!
Provides education and insight for women of all ages who want to under-stand the cyclical nature of their hormone cycle and its influence on their lives. http://www.holyhormones.com

The Healthy Breast Program
This holistic program provides a naturopathic protocol for preventing and treating breast cancer. The program is designed to educate and provide support to women interested in maintaining or improving the health of their breasts. http://www.healthybreastprogram.on.ca

Traditional Chinese Medicine World Foundation
This site explores an approach based on traditional Chinese medicine (TCM) to help regain your natural healing ability and offers a detailed self-care plan to help prevent and speed recovery from breast cancer. http://www.breastcancer.com

Endocrine Disruptors Educational Websites

Children's Health Environmental Coalition
CHEC's mission is to inform about preventable health and development problems caused by exposures to toxic substances in homes, schools and communities and to encourage the public to take action to protect children against these toxic threats. http://www.checnet.org

e.hormone
The e.hormone web site, is a central conduit providing accurate, timely information and educational resources at the cutting edge of environmental signaling research. http://e.hormone.tulane.edu/ehormone.html

Our Stolen Future
The home for the authors of Our Stolen Future, providing regular updates about the cutting edge of science related to endocrine disruption. http://www.ourstolenfuture.org

PANNA (Pesticide Action Network North America)
Links local and international consumer, labor, health, environment and agriculture groups into an international citizens' action network. This network also challenges the global proliferation of pesticides and defends basic rights to health and environmental quality.
http://www.panna.org

Safe 2 Use
Provides education information on toxic chemicals and pesticides.
http://www.safetouse.com

The Children's Environmental Health Network
A national multi-disciplinary organization whose mission is to protect the fetus and the child from environmental health hazards and promote a healthy environment. http://www.cehn.org

The Invisible Gardener
Offers alternatives to chemicals for the natural home, organic gardener, and organic farmer. http://www.invisiblegardener.com

The National Environmental Trust
A non-profit, non-partisan organization established to inform citizens about environmental problems and how they affect our health and quality of life. http://environet.policy.net

The Toxic-free Foundation
A leading resource on the possible toxic ingredients used in personal care, household, baby and pet products.
http://toxicfree.org

References

Part 1
Chapter 2

1. American Cancer Society, Cancer Facts & Figures, 2002

2. Futreal PA, Liu Q, Shattuck-Eidens, D. et al. A Strong candidate for the breast and ovarian cancer susceptibility gene BRCA1. Science 1994; 266:66-71

3. Breast Cancer Research Advance: Same Gene, Depending on Mutation, Can Fight or Cause Tumors, San Francisco Chronicle, March 1, 1996

4. Love, Susan, MD, Dr. Susan Love's Breast Book, Addison-Wesley Publish Company, USA 1994, p.146

5. .Sherman, Janette, M.D., The Delicate Balance of Life, Taylor & Francis, New York 2000 p.6

6. Epstein, Samuel, M.D., Breast Cancer Prevention Program, Macmillan, New York, p.8

Chapter 7

1. http://www.ourstolenfuture.org/Commentary/News/2001-press.htm

Chapter 8

1. Wolff, M., P. Toniolo, E. Lee, M. Rivera, N. Dubin (1993). Blood levels of organochlorines residues and risk of breast cancer. Journal of the National Cancer Institute. 85: (8): 648-652

Chapter 9

1. http://www.ourstolenfuture.org/NewScience/ubiquitous/ubiquitous.htm

Chapter 11

1. http://www.ourstolenfuture.org/Commentary/DD/2001-1012DDhumanitycrisis.htm

Part 2

Chapter 1

1. Berkson, D. Lindsay, Hormone Deception, Contemporary Books, Chicago, IL. 2000, p.82

2. Ibid, p.89

3. op.cit, p.109

Chapter 2

1. Steingraber, Sandra, Having Faith, Perseus Publishing, Cambridge, Mass, 2001, p.34

2. Environment Health Perspectives Supplement 3, Vol. 110 (June 2002), pp.441-449

3. Greenpeace, Poisoning the Future: Impact of Endocrine Disrupting Chemicals on Wild life and Human Health, October 1997 p.23

Chapter 3

1. http://www.marshfieldclinic.org/mc/releases/details.asp?id=2391

2. Salam, MT, Y-F Li, B Langholz and FD Gilliland. 2003. Early Life Environmental Risk Factors for Asthma: Findings from the Children's Health Study. Environmental Health Perspectives. doi:10.1289/ehp.6662 Online 9 December 2003.

3. Latini,G , C de Felice, G Presta, A del Vecchio, I Paris, F Ruggieri, and P Mazzeo. 2003. In utero exposure to di-(2-ethylhexyl)-phthalate and human pregnancy duration .Environmental Health Perspectives, on line 19 August 2003 .

4. http://www.ewg.org/reports/mothersmilk/es.php

5. Johnson, MD, N Kenney, A Stoica, L Hilakiva-Clarke, B Singh, G Chepkko, R Clarke, PF Sholler, AA Lirio, C Foss, R Reiter, B Trock, S Paik and MB Marin. 2003. Cadmium mimics the in vivo effects of estrogen in the uterus and mammary gland .Nature Medicine, online 13 July 2003 .

6. Schreinemachers, DM. 2003. Birth Malformations and Other Adverse Perinatal Outcomes in Four U.S. Wheat - Producing States .Environmental Health Perspectives 111:1259-1264 .

7. http://www.ourstolenfuture.org/Commentary/News/2003/2003-0404-EST-nitrateedc.html

8. Hunt, PA, KE Koehler, M Susiarjo, CA Hodges, A Ilagan, RC Voigt, S Thomas, BF Thomas and TJ Hassold. 2003. Bisphenol A exposure causes meiotic aneuploidy in the female mouse .Current Biology 13: 546-553

Chapter 4

1. http://www.naturalchoicejournal.com/Articles/articles/Breastcancer-Healthoct.htm

Chapter 5

1. http://www.mercola.com/fcgi/pf/2001/jun/13/soy_formula.htm

2. http://www.soyonlineservice.co.nz/home.htm

3. C Irvine, et al, "The Potential Adverse Effects of Soybean Phytoestrogens in Infant Feeding," New Zealand Medical Journal , May 24, 1995, Page 318.

4. Policy Statement of Royal College of Australian Physicians http://www.mercola.com/2001/sep/22/soy_protein_formula_policy.htm

5. http://www.soyonlineservice.co.nz/home.htm

Chapter 6

1. Environmental Medicine: Excerpts from Articles on Current Toxicity, Solvents, Pesticides and Heavy Metals, Townsend Letter for Doctors and Patient, Jan, 2001 by Walter J. Crinnion

2. ibid

3. Ma, X, PA Buffler, RB Gunier, G Dahl, MT Smith, K Reinier and P Reynolds. 2002. Critical Windows of Exposure to Household Pesticides and Risk of Childhood Leukemia .Environmental Health Perspectives 110:955-960 .

4. http://www.checnet.org/healthehouse/education/articles-detail.asp?Main_ID=439

5. Doris Rapp, MD, Our Toxic World: A Wake Up Call ,Environmental Medical Research Foundation, Buffalo, NY, 2004, P. 232

6. Environmental Working Group, " Warning; Teflon Can Cause Birth Defects and Infertility, " March 2003

7. http://www.cpsc.gov

Chapter 8

1. http://mc.net/~chwalisz/itt-cancer-cosm.htm

2. In Vitro and in Vivo Estrogenicity of UV Screens, Environmental Health Perspectives v.109, n.3, Mar 01

Part 3

Chapter 2

1. Herman-Giddes, ME, EJ Slora, RC Wasserman, CJ Bourdony, MV Bhapkar, GG Koch and CH Hassemeir, 1997, Secondary sexual characteristics and menses in young girls seen in office practice: a study from the Pediatric Research Office Settings Network, Pediatrics 99(4): 505-512

2. Time Magazine, "Teens Before Their Time", October 30, 2000

3. ibid

4. Environmental Health Perspectives, Vol 108, No. 9, Sept 2000, pp 895-900

5. Environmental Health Perspectives, Vol 108, No. 10, Oct 2000, pp 979-982

6. Environmental News Network http://www.enn.com/news/enn-stories/200177

7. Time Magazine, "Teens Before Their Time", October 30, 2000

8. Ramos, JG, J Varayoud, C Sonnenschein, AM Soto, M Muñoz de Toro and EH Luque. 2001. Prenatal Exposure to Low Doses of Bisphenol A Alters the Periductal Stroma and Glandular Cell Function in the Rat Ventral Prostate. Biology of Reproduction 65: 1271–1277.

9. http://ehp.niehs.nih.gov/members/1994/102-8/birnbaum-full.html

10. Blount BC, MJ Silva, SP Caudill, LL Needham, JL Pirkle, EJ Sampson, GW Lucier, RJ Jackson, JW Brock. 2000. Levels of seven urinary phthalate metabolites in a human reference population. Environmental Health Perspectives. 108(10):979-982. October 2000.):979-982. October 2000.

11. Environmental Health Perspectives Volume 108, Number 2 February 2000 http://ehp.niehs.nih.gov/members/2000/108p147-152blanck/blanck-full.html

12. http://www.cwg.org/reports/becutesecrets/ch.2.html

Chapter 3

1. Bueckert, Dennis, Hormone -Treated Beef Thought To Trigger Puberty Sooner, Canadian Press, August 2, 1999

2. Epstein op.cit., p.193

3. Ibid, p.194 Ibid, p.196

Chapter 4

1. Berkson, D. Lindsey, Hormone Deception, Contemporary Book, Chicago, Illinois, p.219

Chapter 5

1. http://www.ncbi.nlm.nih.gov/entrez/query.fcgi?cmd=Retrieve&db=PubMed&list_uids=9168006&dopt=Abstract

2. Schlosser, Eric, Fast Food Nation, Houghton- Mifflin Company, N.Y., N.Y.2001 p.126

Chapter 6

1. Janssen J. P., et. al. Effects of soft drink and table beer consumption on insulin response in normal teenagers and carbohydrate drink in youngsters. Eur J Cancer Prev. 1999;Aug; 8 (4):289-95

2. Schlosser, Eric, op. cit. p.54. Schlosser, Eric, op. cit. p.54

3. Blaylock, Russell L.: Excitotoxins: The Taste that Kills, 1997, Health Press

Chapter 7

1. http://www.hsph.harvard.edu/reviews/transfats.html

Part 4

Chapter 1

1. Seaman, Barbara, The Doctors' Case Against the Pill, Hunter House, USA 1995, P 74.

2. Seaman, ibid p. 225

Chapter 2

1. Grant, Ellen MD, Sexual Chemistry, Reed Consumer Books Ltd., U.K. 1994, p. 38

2. Fertility and Sterility 1998;70:30-34

Chapter 3

1. Seaman, op. cit. 223

2. Seaman Ibid 118

3. Seaman Ibid p.225

4. Seaman Ibid

5. Chilvers C., et al. Oral contraceptives use and breast cancer risk in young women. The Lancet, 1989 6th May 973-982

6. Miller DR, Rosenberg L., et al Breast Cancer before age 45 and oral contraceptive use: new findings, American Journal of Epidemiology. 1989;129(2):269-80,Ma.

7. Romieu I et al., Oral contraceptives and breast cancer. Review and meta-analysis. Cancer . 1990:66(11):2253-63.

8. http://ehp.niehs.nih.gov/roc/toc10.html

9. Wilks, John , A Consumers, Guide to the Pill and Other Drugs, Freedom Publishing Company Pty. Ltd., Australia, 1996, p. 84

10. http://www.niehs.nih.gov/

11. John Lee, MD, Ibid, p.73

Chapter 4

1. Grant, ibid. p.12

2. Naish, Francesca, Natural Fertility, Sally Milner Publications, NSW, Australia, 1991 p. 17

3. Naish, Ibid p. 14-16

4. Seaman, ibid. p. 213

Chapter 6

1 . Brandes L.J., Arron R.J., Bogdanovic R.P.,Tong J., Zsaborniak C.L.F., Hogg G.R.,Warrington R., Fang W., La Bella F.S.,"Stimulation of malignant growth in rodents by antidepressent drugs at clinically relevantdoses", Cancer Res 1992;52(13):3796-3800

2. New England Journal of Medicine, vol. 342,June 29, 2000, p. 2003

Part 5

Chapter 5

1. Pope, Alexandra, The Wild Genie, Sally Milner Publishing, Australia 2001

Chapter 12

1. Honara lee Wolfe: and Bob Flaws, Better Breast Health Naturally With Chinese Medicine, Blue Poppy Press, 1998

2. Dr. Kaur, Sat Dhara, A Call to Women, Quarry Health Books, Ontario, Canada 2001

Index

and the use of 284
and where to purchase 309
Naturopathy 197, 263, 275, 299
Non-Toxic Cleaning Solutions 89, 98, 105

O
Oral contraceptives 39, 43, 166-67, 184-85, 277, 299
Organic foods 19, 155
Organochlorines 41-42, 70

Osteopathy 195, 261, 297
Osteoporosis 165, 172, 231-32
     and estrogen dominance 231
     and The Pill 165
Ovarian cancer 21-22, 32, 49, 74, 117, 178, 260
Ovarian cysts 28, 74, 163-64, 189, 194, 196, 199, 228, 231, 248, 259, 283, 288
Ovaries 4, 31, 119, 165, 172, 187, 189
     and polycystic 163-64, 199
     and sugar 139, 144
     and pearl-colored organs 205-06
Ovulation180, 187, 205, 209, 225, 227, 232, 249, 285
     and luteal phase 217
     and suppression 140, 170
     and zinc deficiencies 179

P
Pancreas 140, 189, 223
Paxil 194
Pelvic Inflammatory Disease (PID) 187
Perimenopause 233
Petrochemicals 70
     and carcinogenic pollutants 38, 95-96, 100-01, 131, 151, 157, 299
Phthalates 48, 51-52, 66, 70, 120, 157
Physicians' Desk Reference 154
     and lupron 113

333